Autonomic Disorders

A Case-Based Approach

Autonomic Disorders

A Case-Based Approach

Paola Sandroni, MD, PhD

Professor of Neurology, Mayo Medical School and Head of the Mayo Autonomic Laboratory, Mayo Clinic, Rochester, MN, USA

Phillip A. Low, MD

Robert D. and Patricia E. Kern Professor of Neurology, Mayo Medical School and previous Chair, Division of Clinical Neurophysiology, Department of Neurology, Mayo Clinic, Rochester, MN, USA. He founded the Mayo Autonomic Laboratory in 1983 and pioneered clinical autonomic testing

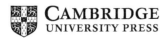

CAMBRIDGE
UNIVERSITY PRESS

CAMBRIDGE
UNIVERSITY PRESS

University Printing House, Cambridge CB2 8BS, United Kingdom

Cambridge University Press is part of the University of Cambridge.

It furthers the University's mission by disseminating knowledge in the pursuit of education, learning and research at the highest international levels of excellence.

www.cambridge.org
Information on this title: www.cambridge.org/9781107400443

© Mayo Foundation for Medical Education and Research 2015

First published 2015

A catalogue record for this publication is available from the British Library

Library of Congress Cataloguing in Publication data
Sandroni, Paola, author.
Autonomic disorders : a case-based approach / Paola Sandroni, Phillip A. Low.
 p. ; cm.
Includes bibliographical references and index.
ISBN 978-1-107-40044-3 (pbk.)
I. Low, Phillip A., author. II. Title.
[DNLM: 1. Autonomic Nervous System Diseases – diagnosis – Atlases. 2. Autonomic Nervous System Diseases – diagnosis – Case Reports. WL 17]
RC407
616.85′69–dc23

2014046182

ISBN 978-1-107-40044-3 Paperback

....

Contents

Preface

This book is designed in atlas format to help physicians to correctly interpret autonomic testing. As such, the illustrative cases and vignettes have been kept very succinct. The goal is to assist not only in pattern recognition, but also to understand the basic pathophysiology underlying various tracings and patterns.

This is not meant to substitute for in-person teaching of course, but as an extension to it.

Other textbooks are available for in-depth information on testing modalities, autonomic function anatomy and physiology, and autonomic disorders.

It was our perception an atlas would fill a specific need currently unmet. Hopefully we succeeded in such endeavor.

Introduction to Tests

Studies cannot be interpreted in the absence of clinical information and testing situations. One can describe the abnormalities, make assumptions, but many may look alike but have very different meanings and implications. Obtaining a detailed history of medications taken (including over-the-counter) prior to testing is crucial as it is vital to have a well-trained technician who can identify technical artifacts, effort or any other patient-related issue that can impact the test quality and meaning.

Note on Figure legends

The testing techniques and physiology have already been detailed in multiple publications and books. Here is simply a key point synopsis to aid the reader.

Deep breathing (a.k.a. metronomic breathing) test: test is performed supine at a breathing rate of 6/min, which generates the largest heart rate variability. The response is generated by the Hering-Breuer reflex (mediated by lung stretch receptors), Bainbridge reflex (mediated right heart filling receptors), and baroreflex activation. Afferent and efferent branches are both vagal, and the signals are processed in the nucleus of the solitary tract. Factors affecting the response include: age, rate of breathing, CO_2 level, presence of primary cardiac or lung pathology, conditions affecting the mechanics of respiration, influence of sympathetic outflow, medications.

Valsalva maneuver: a forced expiration at 40 mmHg for 15 seconds performed supine. The maneuver results in a fall of BP (early phase II) that activates baroreflex. This triggers a sympathetic surge with

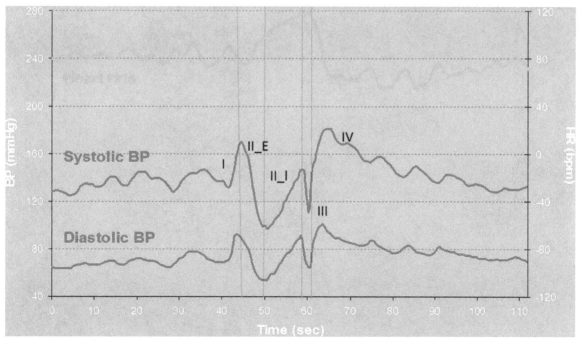

Fig. I.1

peripheral vasoconstriction and tachycardia that generates a BP rise (late phase II), usually with mean BP back to baseline value. At the end of the maneuver, a brief drop in blood pressure occurs (phase III), followed by an overshoot (phase IV). Baroreflex activation blocks the sympathetic outflow and triggers vagal surge, resulting in bradycardia and release of peripheral vasoconstriction (Fig. I.1). Factors affecting the response include: position of the subject, expiratory pressure, duration of effort, age and gender, volume status, medications. Valsalva ratio = maximum/minimum HR. The blood pressure profile should be described, including recovery time (time from the bottom of phase III to return to baseline BP; normal value < 6 seconds) if abnormal.

Tilt test: passive tilt-up for 10 minutes after 20–30 minutes supine baseline. Blood pressure and heart rate are monitored beat-to-beat throughout the studies.

Quantitative sudomotor axon reflex test (QSART): after stable baseline is obtained, acetylcholine is iontophoresed by applying electrical stimulation for 5 minutes, recording continues for 5 minutes more. By activation of axon reflex, sweating occurs. Sweat volume is obtained by integrating the area under the 10 minute curve.

QSART tracings: red = forearm; blue = proximal leg; green = distal leg; yellow = foot. The marks indicate: start of recordings to obtain baseline, acetylcholine injection in capsule, stimulation starts, stimulation ends, recording ends.

Deep breathing (DB), Valsalva maneuver (VM) and tilt tracings: blue = chest strap indicating breathing effort; green = heart rate; red = systolic blood pressure; pink = mean BP; yellow = diastolic BP and expiratory pressure generated during VM. During DB the marks indicate each inspiratory and expiratory act. During VM the marks indicate: patients take deep breath, expiratory effort start, expiratory effort ends. During tilt the marks indicate tilt-up and tilt-down.

Thermoregulatory sweat test (TST): the normally sweating areas are in purple, while the areas with reduced or absent sweat are in yellow. The test utilizes alizarin red as an indicator, which turns from yellow to purple when wet. Actual photos are shown, not the drawings. Reduced sweat is often seen over bony areas, callused skin, stretch marks, scars, and various skin conditions.

Normal examples

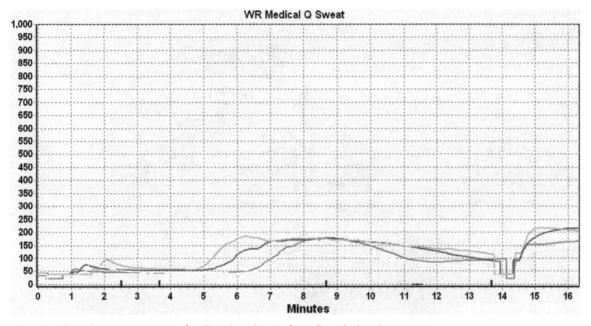

Fig. I.2(a). Normal sweat responses in a female and a male case. Generally, males have larger output.

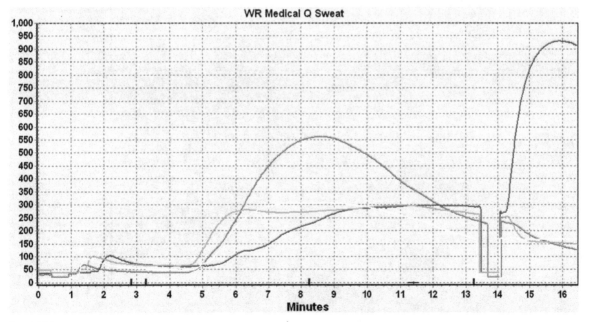

Fig. I.2(b).

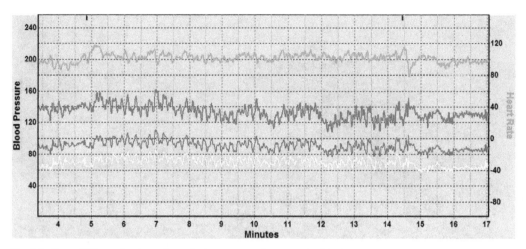

Fig. I.3. Normal tilt: very few hemodynamic changes occur in a normal subject

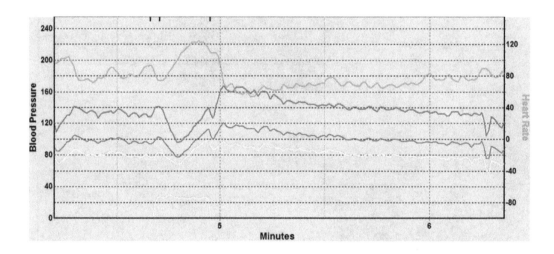

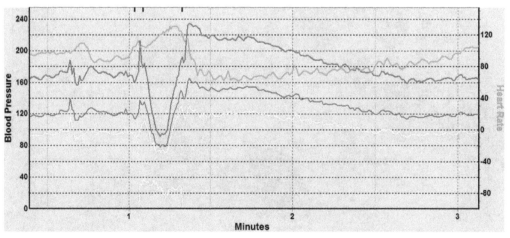

Fig. I.4. Two examples of normal Valsalva profiles: note the robust blood pressure rise during late phase II particularly in the second tracing, induced by a more prominent early phase II and pulse pressure compression suggesting volume contraction. Phase IV is also well demarcated. The heart rate shows a good acceleration during the maneuver followed by a rapid drop below baseline during phase IV.

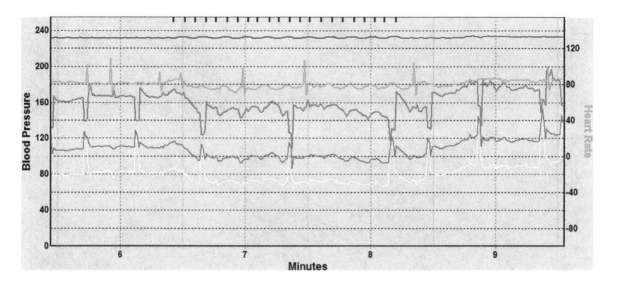

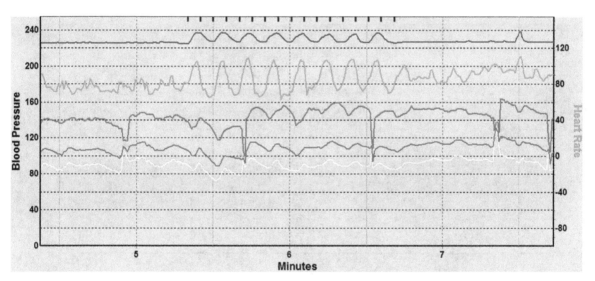

Fig. I.5. Deep breathing profile in an older subject (top) and a younger one: the amplitude of the heart rate oscillations diminishes with age. In comparison, in the young they can be > 40 beats per minute.

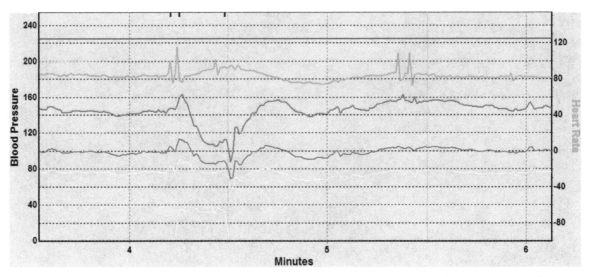

Fig. I.6. Valsalva maneuver in an older subject: late phase II rise may be blunted. It may be expression of mild dysautonomia of aging.

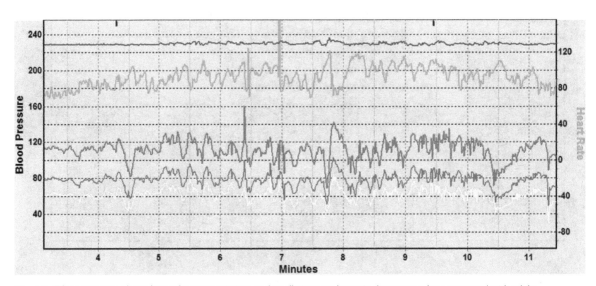

Fig. I.7. Tilt in a young subject: hemodynamic variations and oscillations are larger in the young when compared with adults.

Prodromal possible Lewy body disease

History

A 44-year-old male presented with a history that began at the age of 37 years when he started to experience terrifying nightmares that he acted-out by thrashing his limbs or jumping out of bed. At the age of 42 years he began to complain of increasing light-headedness that worsened over time, resulting in multiple presyncopal episodes. Heat and activity worsen the symptoms. He noticed that he had stopped sweating over most of his body but reported increased sweating over his head. Except for mild constipation and bloating, he had no significant gastrointestinal symptoms. He felt he was not emptying his bladder fully and was experiencing erectile dysfunction not responsive to sildenafil. At the age of 43 years he began to have mild gait unsteadiness with a wide-based gait and frequent stumbling. Speech was unaffected as were his limb movements. There was no unequivocal cognitive difficulty. More recently he had been complaining of profound fatigue.

He had no significant past medical history except for a mild concussion at the age of 19 years. He worked as a welder and reported being exposed to various chemicals, including manganese. He also reported that two of his co-workers were diagnosed with multiple system atrophy.

The remaining history was unremarkable. His medications included midodrine, fludrocortisone, melatonin, and zolpidem.

Examination

Neurologic examination was normal except for a mild deficit on the heel-to-shin test.

Pertinent tests

Complete blood count, routine chemistry analysis, neuroimmunology panel, and thyroid-stimulating hormone-sensitive testing were normal. Plasma norepinephrine level was 116 pg/mL when supine and 204 pg/mL when standing (an inadequate rise considering his orthostatic hypotension). The patient had a urine output of 1600 cm^3 over 24 hours with 203 mEq/L of sodium excretion (suggesting excellent fluid and salt intake).

Polysomnography revealed the presence of REM behavior disorder. Neuropsychometric testing was mildly abnormal, with deficits mainly in auditory verbal learning and memory that were not specific for any neurodegenerative disorder.

Autonomic testing showed that cardiovagal function was mildly reduced (Fig. 1.1), there was abnormal

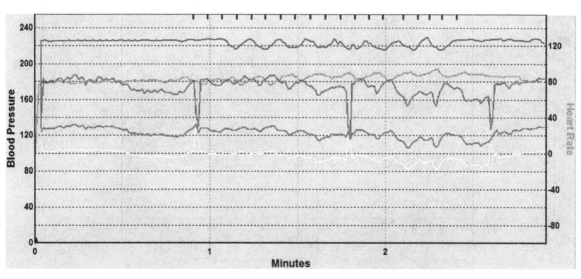

Fig. 1.1 Heart rate response to deep breathing was reduced for age.

vasoconstriction during Valsalva with altered cardiac responses (Fig. 1.2), and identified the presence of orthostatic hypotension (Fig. 1.3). Sweating was only mildly abnormal on both QSART (Fig. 1.4) and TST (Fig. 1.5).

Comments

The case illustrates an example of what is most likely Lewy body disease [DLB] at an early stage.

With such degree of abnormality on autonomic testing, multiple system atrophy [MSA] would have had more anhidrosis. DLB has more autonomic involvement than Parkinson's disease, but less than MSA as a group. Cognitive abnormalities are typically absent in MSA. There is no evidence that manganese or other toxins can cause DLB or MSA, while it can cause parkinsonism.

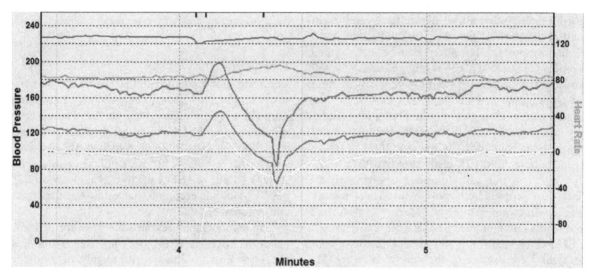

Fig. 1.2 Valsalva maneuver: there is reduced Valsalva ratio, indicating impaired cardiac responses, and the blood pressure profile is abnormal, with absence of late phase II and IV and prolonged recovery time.

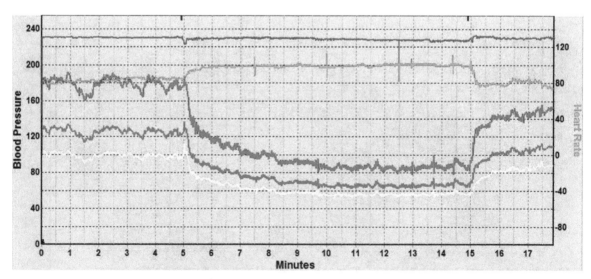

Fig. 1.3 Tilt study showed presence of orthostatic hypotension with attenuated cardiac responses.

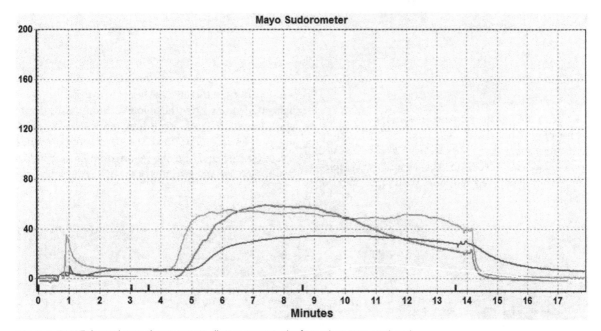

Fig. 1.4 QSART showed normal responses in all sites except in the foot, where it was reduced.

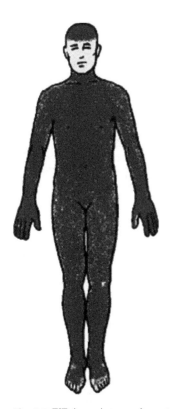

Fig. 1.5 TST showed a normal sweat pattern.

Multiple system atrophy – cerebellar type

History

A 57-year-old female presented with an 18-month history of gait imbalance. She reported an insidious onset and evaluation at her local doctor's office revealed supine hypertension (new for her) as well as asymptomatic orthostatic hypotension. With the start of antihypertensive therapy, she began to experience severe light-headedness. Over the following months, she developed dysarthria, R > L upper-limb tremor, and worsening gait unsteadiness. Next she began to experience severe bladder urgency. She reported no change in her bowel pattern or sweating capacity. Although she

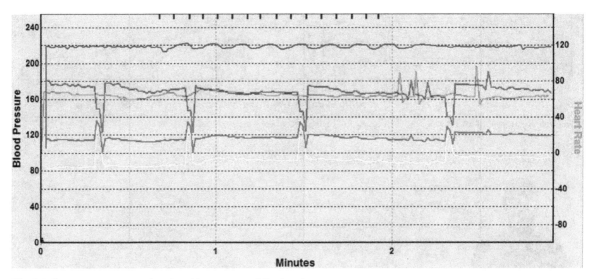

Fig. 2.1 Heart rate response to deep breathing was essentially absent.

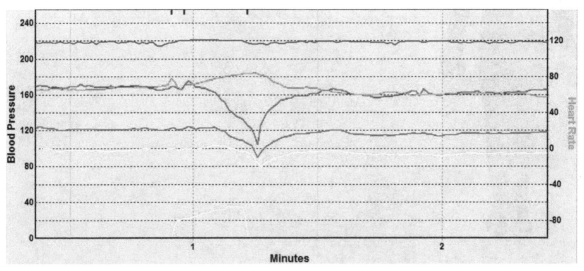

Fig. 2.2 Valsalva maneuver: there is reduced Valsalva ratio, indicating impaired cardiac responses, and the blood pressure profile is abnormal, with absence of late phase II and IV and prolonged recovery time.

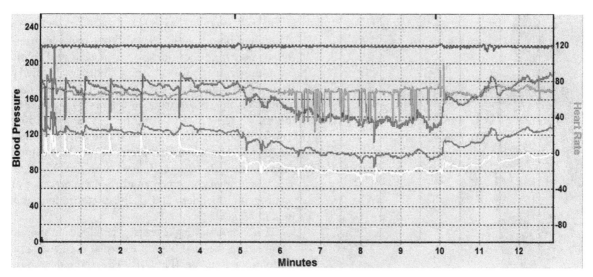

Fig. 2.3 Tilt study showed presence of supine hypertension, orthostatic hypotension and no compensatory cardiac response.

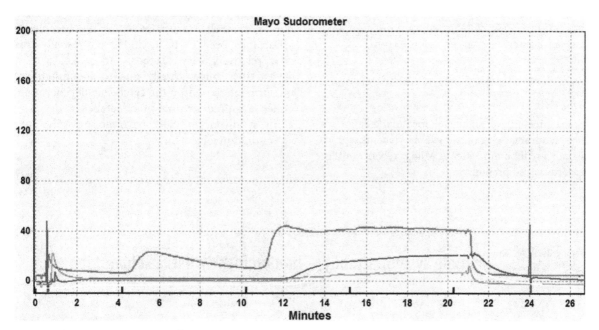

Fig. 2.4 QSART responses were normal.

described features suggestive of REM sleep behavior disorder [RBD] and stridor, a sleep study confirmed disordered breathing and presence of myoclonus but no RBD. Her motor performance continued to rapidly decline so that she was wheelchair bound and dependent in all her activities of daily living at presentation in our facility. A trial of carbidopa-levodopa started by the local doctor was of no benefit.

She had no significant past medical, social, or family history. Her medications included midodrine, pyridostigmine, and fludrocortisone, which were only marginally beneficial.

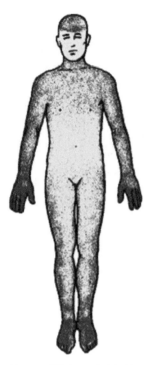

Examination

The examination was significant for a marked pancerebellar syndrome with ataxic eye movements, speech, and gait and limb movements. Mild cerebellar outflow tremor was also present.

Pertinent tests

Complete blood count, electrolytes, neuroimmunology panel, endocrine testing, plasma and urine immunoelectrophoresis, and routine chemistry tests were normal. Heavy metal screen was negative. Norepinephrine level was 517 and 569 pg/mL respectively supine and standing (normal supine level but no rise on standing, which is abnormal in presence of orthostatic hypotension).

The urodynamic study confirmed the presence of neurogenic bladder and self-catheterization was recommended.

Autonomic-testing revealed generalized autonomic failure (Figs 2.1–2.3) but with normal postganglionic sudomotor function (Fig. 2.4). TST showed marked anhidrosis, thus suggesting a preganglionic lesion (Fig. 2.5).

Comments

This is a classic example of multiple system atrophy – cerebellar type [MSA-C]. Paraneoplastic syndromes need to be excluded but usually this is a relatively easy diagnosis to make, with a devastating course chiefly due to the functional impairment caused by the cerebellar degeneration. Other acquired or inherited cerebellar degeneration syndromes usually have no or only mild autonomic involvement.

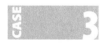

Multiple system atrophy – predominantly parkinsonian type

History

A 53-year-old male presented initially at the age of 43 years with a left-leg limp. His gait became slow with small shuffling steps. He then developed clumsiness of the left hand. He did not fall initially. At age of 45 years he was started on Sinemet with a definite improvement in his symptoms. His parkinsonism progressed and at the age of 48 years he began to fall and now he falls on an almost daily basis. His voice has become progressively softer. He had not had rest tremor at any time throughout his illness. He had a long-standing, very mild, postural tremor. There was no clear asymmetry to his symptoms of bradykinesia and rigidity. He continued to experience benefit from the Sinemet. He was taking this four times a day and was aware of wearing-off phenomena towards the end of each dose. He would develop episodes of freezing and become more bradykinetic. This improved with the addition of amantadine. He denied any dyskinesias or dystonias.

He also developed urinary incontinence beginning at the age of 47 years. He had both frequency and urgency. His urinary incontinence was not simply related to his impaired mobility. He had incomplete bladder emptying and often has to void twice within 10 minutes. He wore continence pads. He had not required urinary catheterization. He has had some relief in the early stages with oxybutynin with respect to his urgency but the benefit had since worn off. He was able to void without applying abdominal pressure, but he felt that he voids more completely if he passed a bowel motion at the same time. He has had long-standing constipation with hard stools. He would occasionally have fecal incontinence which he related more to his impaired mobility. He did not have early satiety or postprandial vomiting. He has had erectile dysfunction since the age of 50 years. With the aid of sildenafil, he could achieve an erection but was unable to ejaculate. He had not noticed any change in his sweating. It was unclear whether he had symptoms of orthostatic hypotension. On several occasions after a meal on standing up, he had felt unbalanced and had fallen over. However, this had not been associated with any preceding dizziness,

light-headedness, or faintness. His neurologist had not documented a significant postural drop in the past. Also noted was mild cognitive slowing and obsessive-compulsive disorder-type behavior.

A PET scan done at the age of 52 years was interpreted as abnormal and consistent with Parkinson's disease rather than multiple system atrophy.

Examination

His examination was consistent with a rigid parkinsonian syndrome of moderate severity.

Pertinent tests

Complete blood count, electrolytes, neuroimmunology panel, endocrine testing, plasma and urine immunoelectrophoresis, and routine chemistry tests were unremarkable.

Plasma catecholamines revealed a supine norepinephrine level of 81 and a standing level of 151 pg/mL (low supine level with inadequate rise on standing).

His autonomic study showed presence of borderline cardiac responses (Figs 3.1 and 3.2), with borderline orthostatic hypotension (Fig. 3.3) and postganglionic sudomotor impairment (Fig. 3.4). His TST showed 90% anhidrosis (Fig. 3.5).

Follow-up

One year later, the patient returned for reassessment. At that point he required an indwelling urinary

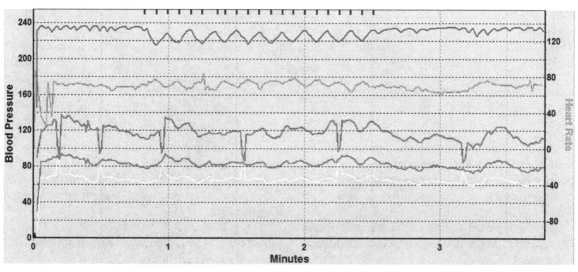

Fig. 3.1 Heart rate response to deep breathing was mildly reduced for age.

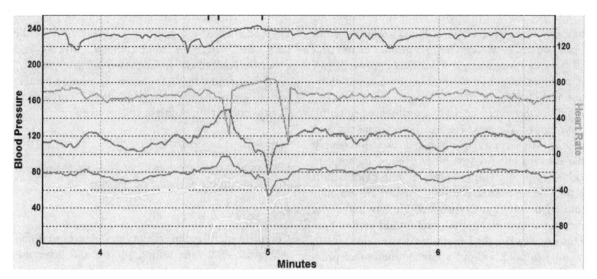

Fig. 3.2 Valsalva maneuver: there is reduced Valsalva ratio, indicating impaired cardiac responses, and the blood pressure profile is abnormal, with absence of late phase II, reduced phase IV, and prolonged recovery time.

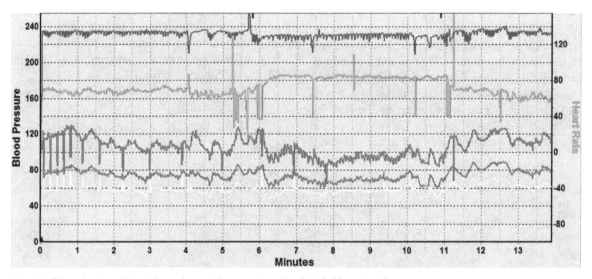

Fig. 3.3 Tilt study showed borderline orthostatic hypotension with relatively blunted cardiac responses.

catheter and his motor symptoms had progressed. On examination he had mild ataxia and upgoing toes, besides mild worsening of his preexistent parkinsonian syndrome. No further cognitive changes were noted.

His wife reported occasional nocturnal stridor, and questionable episodes suggestive of REM behavior disorder.

A TST and autonomic study were repeated after withholding oxybutinin for 2 weeks (first time the test was withheld for 36 hours); although still abnormal, the abnormalities were much less pronounced than the prior year (Fig. 3.6).

The patient died 3 years later and autopsy confirmed the diagnosis of multiple system atrophy, with diffuse alpha-synuclein deposition.

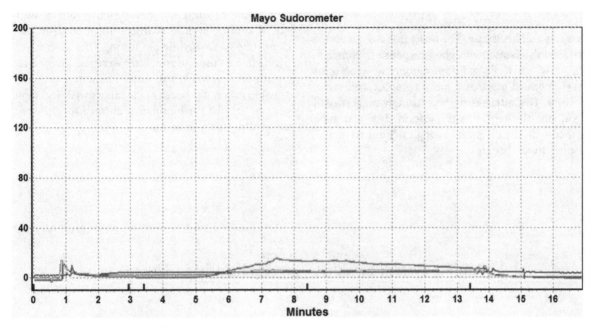

Fig. 3.4 QSART responses were reduced or absent for all sites.

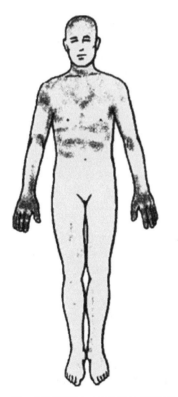

Fig. 3.5 TST showed global anhidrosis, but the patient had taken his last dose of oxybutynin 36 hours prior to the study.

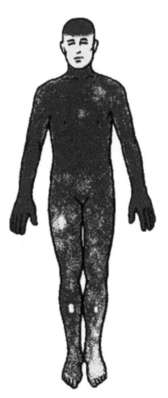

Fig. 3.6 TST showed "improvement." In reality it was simply due to the fact the patient withheld his medication for 2 weeks prior to testing.

Comment

This was a difficult case. The onset initially suggested Parkinson's disease, with good response to Sinemet. The early onset of significant autonomic symptoms clearly pointed towards a more complex syndrome, however. The initial testing was strongly suggestive of MSA, but the repeat tests performed 1 year later clashed with the diagnosis owing to "improvement," despite clinical progression.

Caveat: Medications can seriously affect autonomic studies, even after discontinuation, if insufficient time is allowed before testing. This case is still perplexing as the abnormalities were less severe than usually seen in MSA, but motor and autonomic progression may not proceed at the same speed, and some systems may be predominantly affected (in this case, the genitourinary system).

4 Multiple system atrophy – predominantly parkinsonism

History

A 46-year-old female presented with a 3-year history of urinary incontinence and retention, for which she was treated conservatively at first. Later a sacral nerve stimulator was implanted but this was unsuccessful and she had recently resorted to self-catheterization. Over time she had also developed increasingly severe neck ache and orthostatic light-headedness, gait difficulties due to bradykinesia, and freezing episodes. She reported only occasional hand tremor, micrographia, and cognitive slowing. She had no gastrointestinal symptoms except nausea, which was thought to be medication related. Her husband described episodes suggestive of REM behavior disorder over 10 years prior to presentation, but stated they had improved. She had a history of depression, for which she was monitored by a psychiatrist.

There was no family history of neurologic disorders. There was no history of toxic exposure or other significant medical history except for depression as noted above.

Examination

The patient had some mild deficits on mental status testing, but she was very anxious during the exam and had taken opiates to control her neck pain. She had clear findings of parkinsonism with hypomimia, hypophonia, cogwheel rigidity, generalized

bradykinesia, shuffling gait, and mild unsteadiness. She had a tendency to fall to the right even in a sitting position. No tremor was present. Reflexes were diffusely brisk, with bilateral positive Babinski and Chaddock's signs. Orthostatic hypotension was present.

Pertinent tests

Extensive testing failed to identify a treatable cause for the patient's condition. Complete blood count, electrolytes, neuroimmunology panel, endocrine testing, plasma and urine immunoelectrophoresis, and routine chemistry tests were normal. Heavy metal screen was negative.

Plasma catecholamines showed a norepinephrine level of 155 supine and 186 pg/mL standing, which is a very small rise considering the severity of her orthostatic hypotension.

Brain MRI revealed mild atrophy for age and MRI of the cervical spine showed marked degenerative changes without clear intrinsic cord abnormalities.

An autonomic screen showed mild cardiovagal (Fig. 4.1), severe cardiovascular adrenergic (Figs 4.2 and 4.3) and moderate postganglionic sudomotor impairment (Fig. 4.4).

TST showed significant anhidrosis (50%) (Fig. 4.5) consistent with a central autonomic disorder.

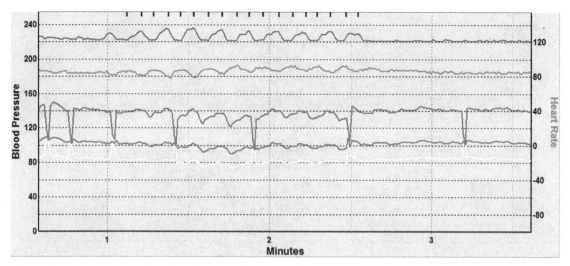

Fig. 4.1 Heart rate response to deep breathing was mildly reduced for age.

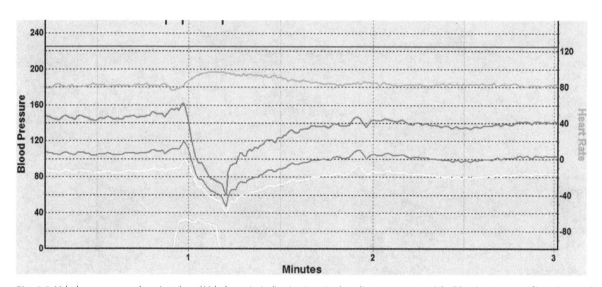

Fig. 4.2 Valsalva maneuver: there is reduced Valsalva ratio, indicating impaired cardiac responses, and the blood pressure profile is abnormal, with absence of late phase II and IV and markedly prolonged recovery time.

Overnight oximetry showed no convincing evidence of disordered breathing.

Follow-up

Despite aggressive symptomatic management, which included a trial of carbidopa-levodopa, pressor agents, physical and occupational therapy, the patient declined very rapidly and became essentially bed-bound within 1 year.

Comments

This case represents a particularly malignant course of multiple system atrophy predominantly parkinsonism [MSA-P] that started at an unusually young age. The history of REM behavior disorder, the relentless progression of autonomic and motor symptoms, and the test results left little doubt on the presence of a neurodegenerative condition.

17

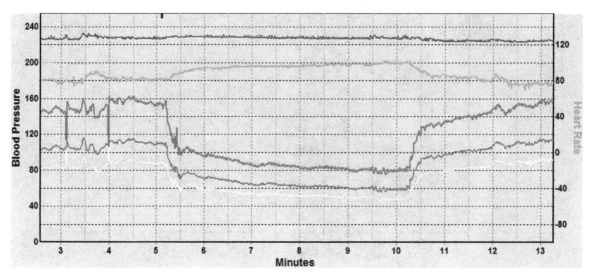

Fig. 4.3 Tilt study showed presence of orthostatic hypotension with attenuated cardiac responses

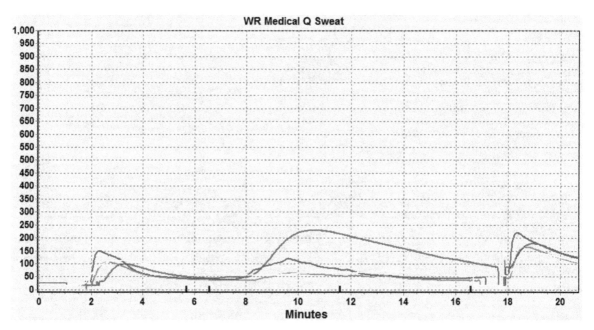

Fig. 4.4 QSART responses were reduced at the distal leg and foot sites.

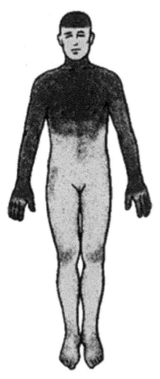

Fig. 4.5 TST showed anhidrosis in the lower half of the body.

 ## Pure autonomic failure

History

A 57-year-old male presented for reassessment and management of his symptoms of light-headedness, impaired sweating, and erectile dysfunction. These have been present (albeit less marked) for over 16 years. Over the years, his symptoms progressed slowly and he developed sicca complex with dry eyes and mouth. He reported no significant bladder dysfunction and occasional alternating bowel habits. He has no other deficits.

As his symptoms evolved slowly he had been able to compensate and develop strategies to cope with them, thus remaining fully functional.

He has no other medical problem. His medications have been fludrocortisone, pyridostigmine, and midodrine for many years with only minimal changes in doses over time.

Examination

The neurologic examination was normal.

Pertinent tests

Extensive testing failed to identify a treatable cause for this patient's condition. His blood tests, including complete blood count, electrolytes and routine chemistry group, thyroid-stimulating hormone-sensitive testing, plasma and urine immunoelectrophoresis, and neuroimmunology panel were unremarkable. Heavy metal screen was negative.

Plasma norepinephrine levels were barely detectable (14 pg/mL) with no changes in standing position.

Autonomic screen: severe global failure, affecting cardiovagal, cardiovascular adrenergic and postganglionic sudomotor functions (Figs 5.1–5.4).

TST showed global anhidrosis (100%) (Fig. 5.5).

Comments

This is a classic case of pure autonomic failure [PAF], with global autonomic failure in absence of any other nervous system involvement, either central or peripheral. The very low plasma norepinephrine when supine is characteristic of this disorder, although can be seen in severe autonomic ganglioneuropathies. The long, slow history, and the absence of other neurologic symptoms except for the autonomic ones, differentiate it from multiple system atrophy [MSA]. Nonetheless, this condition is a synucleinopathy and we have seen cases evolve into MSA or Lewy body disease even after many years.

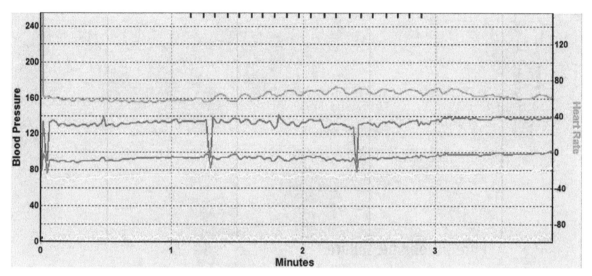

Fig. 5.1 Heart rate response to deep breathing was reduced for age.

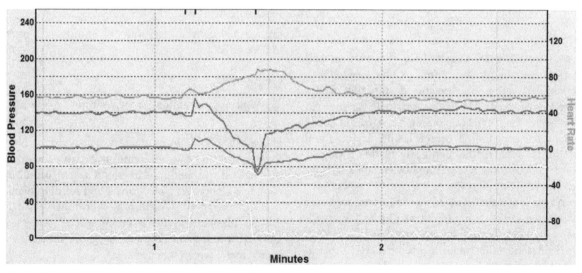

Fig. 5.2 Valsalva maneuver: there is reduced Valsalva ratio for age, indicating impaired cardiac responses, and the blood pressure profile is abnormal, with absence of late phase II and IV and prolonged recovery time.

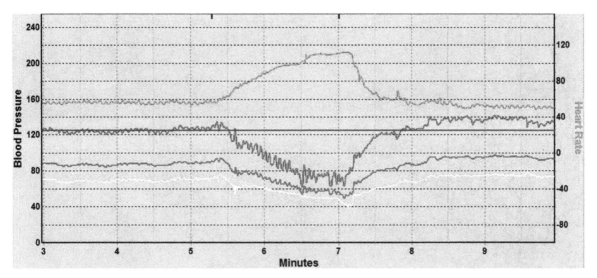

Fig. 5.3 Tilt study showed severe orthostatic hypotension with a valid compensatory cardioacceleration, albeit still unable to sustain the blood pressure.

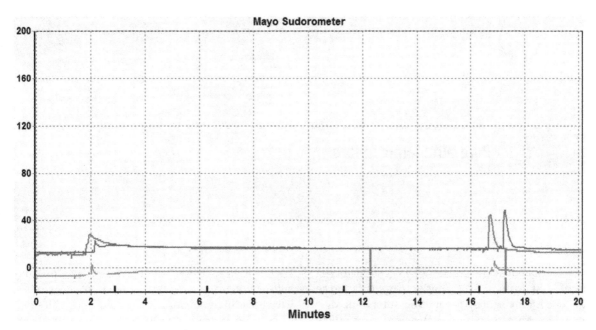

Fig. 5.4 QSART responses were absent for all sites.

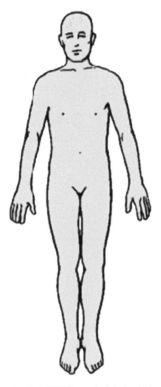

Fig. 5.5 TST showed global anhidrosis.

 **Pure autonomic failure**

History

A 55-year-old male presented with a 2-year history of erectile dysfunction. One year prior to presentation he developed fairly acutely generalized autonomic dysfunction, with orthostatic hypotension, early satiety and bloating, alternating bowel pattern, weight loss, heat intolerance, and bladder dysfunction. During his evaluation, prostate cancer had been incidentally found and treated successfully, with no changes in his bladder or sexual complaints.

He had no other significant medical problem.

Examination

The neurologic exam was normal.

Pertinent tests

He was tested extensively to rule out amyloidosis and autoimmune causes. Complete blood count, electrolytes, neuroimmunology panel, endocrine testing, plasma and urine immunoelectrophoresis, and routine chemistry tests were normal. Plasma norepinephrine was 33 pg/mL supine and 54 pg/mL standing.

Autonomic screen showed generalized autonomic failure (Figs 6.1–6.4).

TST showed global anhidrosis of 97% (Fig. 6.5).

Gastrointestinal transit study showed slightly accelerated gastric emptying and small bowel transit.

Subsequently the patient suffered a bout of diverticulitis requiring partial colectomy, with excellent outcome.

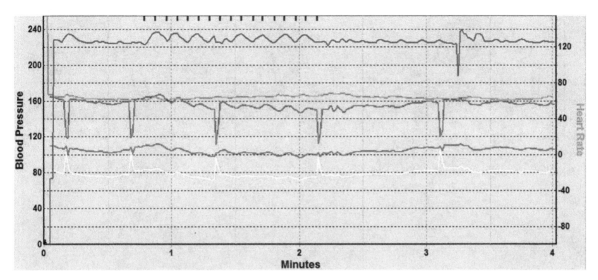

Fig. 6.1 Heart rate response to deep breathing was essentially absent.

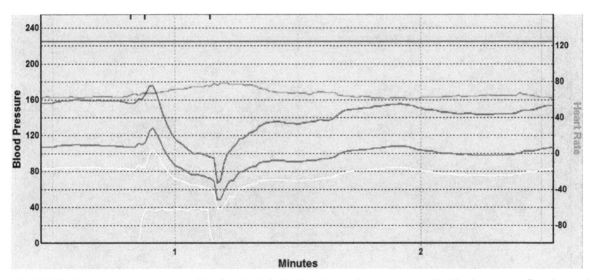

Fig. 6.2 Valsalva maneuver: there is reduced Valsalva ratio, indicating impaired cardiac responses, and the blood pressure profile is abnormal, with absence of late phase II and IV and prolonged recovery time.

Follow-up

At 3 years re-check, he was clinically stable, with symptomatic management for orthostatic hypotension being partially successful. He has developed worsening supine hypertension, as documented in his Holter monitoring (Fig. 6.6), requiring short-acting medication at night (Procardia). He had developed no symptoms or signs suggestive of evolution into multiple system atrophy [MSA] or diffuse Lewy body disease [DLB].

Comments

This is similar to the preceding case. Also, once such diagnosis is established it is important not to overlook other medical conditions that may be causing or contributing to some symptoms, in this case, prostate cancer and diverticulitis were responsible at least in part for some of the patient's complaints.

Supine hypertension can become severe enough to require medication at bedtime, when

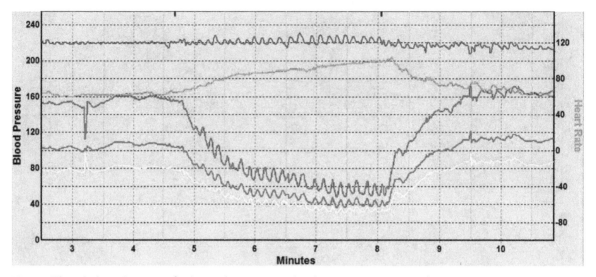

Fig. 6.3 Tilt study showed presence of orthostatic hypotension and inadequate compensatory cardiac response.

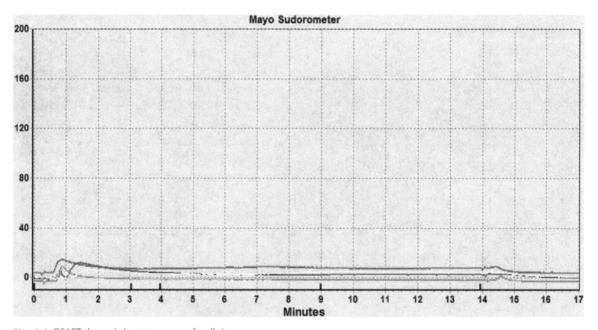

Fig. 6.4 QSART showed absent responses for all sites.

elevation of the head of the bed is not sufficient anymore. It is best to use short-acting agents and warn the patient of the risk of hypotension if they need to get out of bed during the night. Besides the intrinsic risks of hypertension, another problem it causes is nocturnal diuresis, which may significantly disrupt the patient's sleep and result in volume contraction by morning, hence worsening orthostatic hypotension upon awakening.

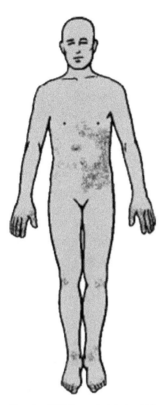

Fig. 6.5 TST showed global anhidrosis.

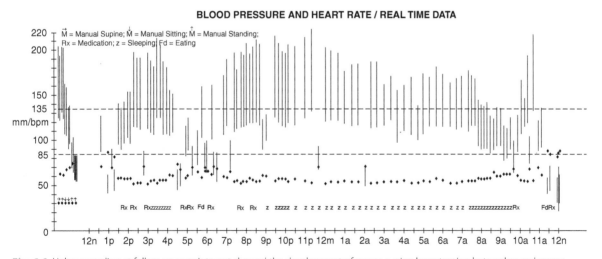

Fig. 6.6 Holter recording at follow-up appointment showed the development of severe supine hypertension but unchanged severe orthostatic hypotension.

CASE 7   Acute autonomic ganglionopathy

History

A 55-year-old female with a 5-year history of diabetes type II in excellent control, presented 6 months after she contracted a flu-like illness with vomiting, nausea, diarrhea, as well as upper respiratory symptoms, and soon thereafter she developed orthostatic intolerance with frank orthostatic hypotension and syncopal episodes. She also complained of a very dry mouth, blurry vision, and possibly decreased sweat. She had a poor appetite. She also developed symptoms that suggested early satiety, and she lost about 50 lb since then. Also, she developed quite severe constipation. She had no other neurologic or systemic symptoms.

Examination

She had dilated pupils that reacted poorly to light. She had dry mucosae and dry skin. The examination was otherwise normal. Specifically, there was no evidence of peripheral neuropathy.

Pertinent tests

Complete blood count, electrolytes, and chemistry group were normal except for plasma glucose =

144mg/dL and HbA1C = 7.3%. Monoclonal protein studies were normal. Neuroimmunology panel showed a positive acetylcholine ganglionic receptor autoantibody (AchR-Ab) titer of 13 (normal < 0.02 nmol/L).

Norepinephrine levels were = 29 pg/mL supine and 52 pg/mL standing.

Autonomic study showed severe, generalized autonomic failure (Figs 7.1–7.4) and TST demonstrated widespread patchy anhidrosis of the lower limbs, lower trunk, and to a lesser extent of the upper limbs (Fig. 7.5).

Comment

This is a classic example of acute autonomic ganglionopathy [AAG]. The significant cholinergic dysfunction is a prominent feature of this disorder and anticholinergic intoxication or botulism should be excluded. Higher titer is usually associated with greater clinical cholinergic impairment. Even when the history is strongly suggestive, some patients may be antibody negative, but still be responsive to immunotherapy. This case had the potential confounding factor of diabetes, but she had been in excellent control and it would have been very unlikely for her to develop such acute autonomic dysfunction. On the

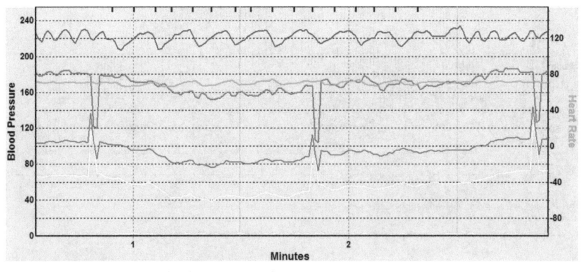

26   Fig. 7.1 Heart rate responses to deep breathing were reduced for age.

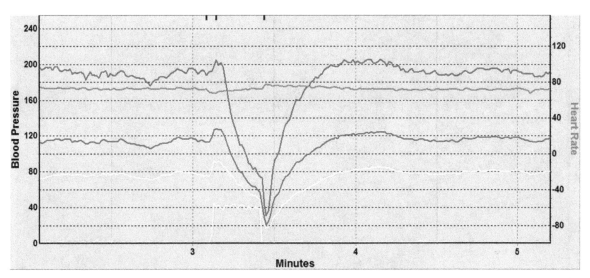

Fig. 7.2 Valsalva maneuver: there is markedly reduced Valsalva ratio, indicating impaired cardiac responses, and the blood pressure profile is abnormal, with absence of late phase II, reduced/absent phase IV and prolonged recovery time.

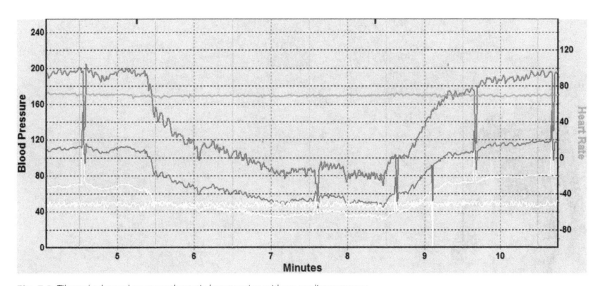

Fig. 7.3 Tilt study showed severe orthostatic hypotension with no cardiac response.

other hand, some diabetic patients, usually poorly controlled type I with evidence of complications, may present with rapid deterioration, mimicking AAG. An autoimmune mechanism may still be involved (other than the AchR autoantibody) and immunotherapy may thus be at least partially effective, at least in part.

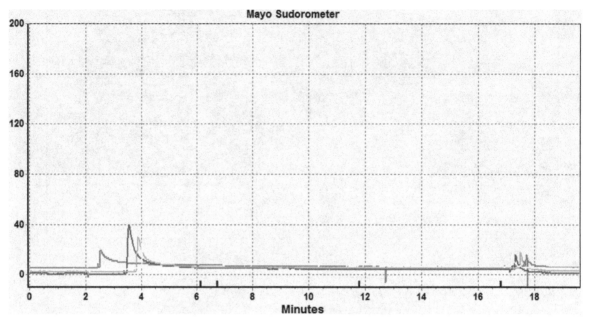

Fig. 7.4 QSART responses were absent for all sites.

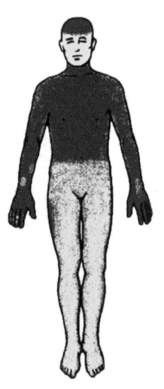

Fig. 7.5 TST showed anhidrosis over the lower half of the body with patchy anhidrosis of the upper limbs.

Acute autonomic ganglionopathy

History

A 49-year-old male, previously healthy, presented for evaluation of subacute onset of nausea, inability to void (requiring self-catheterization), erectile dysfunction, dry mouth, loss of sweating, and syncope. He subsequently developed ileus requiring hospitalization. He was treated empirically with 5 days of intravenous immunoglobulin (IVIG) with only limited improvement. He lost 45 lb over 3 months unintentionally due to this illness.

The rest of his history was non-contributory.

Examination

The neurologic examination was normal. Dry skin was noted.

Pertinent tests

Extensive laboratory tests (complete blood count, electrolytes, neuroimmunology panel, endocrine testing, plasma and urine immunoelectrophoresis, and routine chemistry tests) were unremarkable, including a negative AChR antibody. Fat aspirate was negative for amyloid.

Norepinephrine levels were 91 pg/mL supine and 218 pg/mL standing, which was an inadequate rise considering his profound orthostatic hypotension.

The autonomic screen revealed the presence of generalized autonomic failure, consistent with a severe autonomic neuropathy or ganglionopathy (Figs 8.1–8.4).

TST showed global anhidrosis (Figs 8.5(a) and (b)).

The patient was diagnosed with seronegative acute autonomic ganglionopathy [AAG] and started on a prolonged course of immunotherapy.

At the most recent assessment, 2 years later, he has regained some of his lost weight, has improved significantly with regard to his orthostatic tolerance (Fig 8.6–8.7) – albeit still on symptomatic treatment. Bladder and bowel function have improved but he continues to have severe erectile dysfunction and anhidrosis.

Comment

Seropositive and seronegative AAG may be indistinguishable. Although as a group seropositive cases appear to have more prominent cholinergic failure, this patient had fairly severe cholinergic dysfunction. The temporal profile and negative search for alternate diagnosis was the key in this specific case.

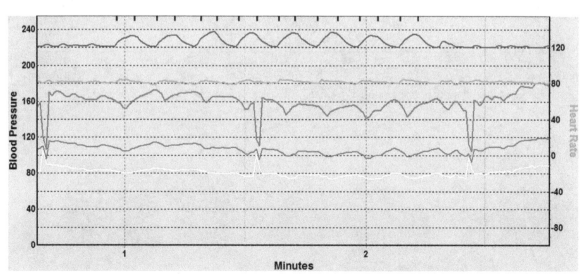

Fig. 8.1 Heart rate response to deep breathing was markedly attenuated for age.

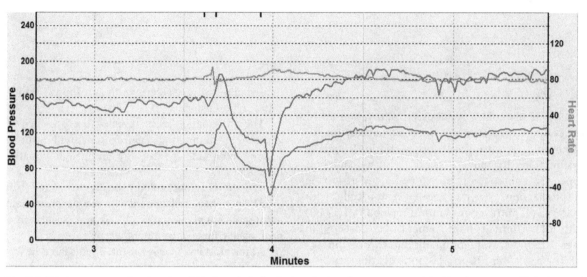

Fig. 8.2 Valsalva maneuver: there is reduced Valsalva ratio, indicating impaired cardiac responses, and the blood pressure profile is abnormal, with absence of late phase II, reduced phase IV, and prolonged recovery time.

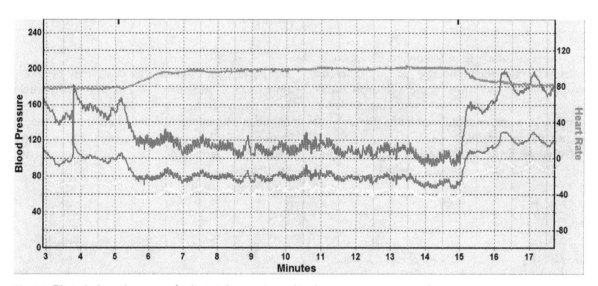

Fig. 8.3 Tilt study showed presence of orthostatic hypotension and inadequate compensatory cardiac response.

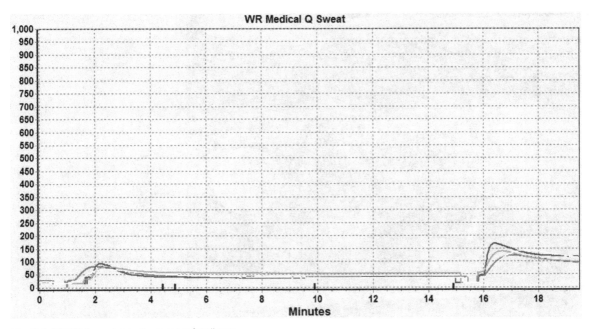

Fig. 8.4 QSART showed absent responses for all sites.

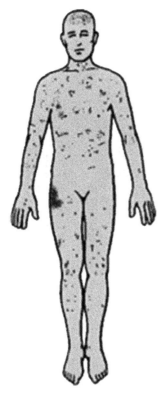

Fig. 8.5(a) TST showed global anhidrosis, with only small islands of preserved sweat.

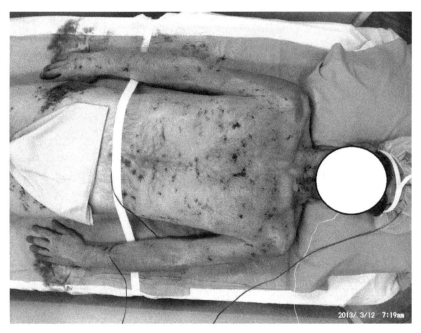

Fig. 8.5(b) Actual photo taken at the end of TST.

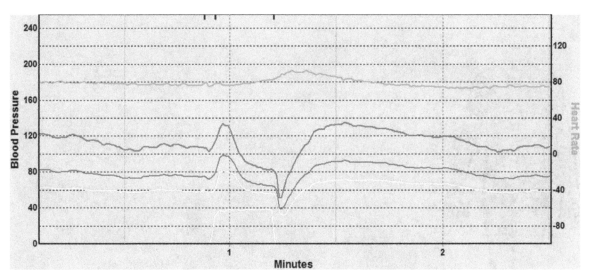

Fig. 8.6 Follow-up Valsalva study showed some improvement in blood pressure recovery time and phase IV.

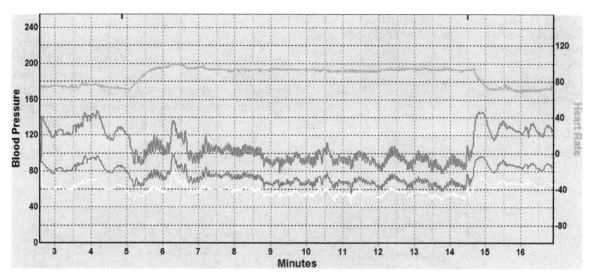

Fig. 8.7 Tilt study showed less severe orthostatic hypotension and mild improvement of cardiac responses when compared with the first study.

9 Acute autoimmune autonomic ganglionopathy

History

A 66-year-old female presented with a history of fecal urgency, without incontinence, immediately after eating or drinking that started 8 years ago. Stools were loose, not black, nor bloody. There was no abdominal pain. At the time she was under some stress and she did not pay much attention to the condition, which anyway resolved in 48 hours.

Since then she has been complaining of constipation with bowel movements occurring every 3 days, with passage of hard, small stools. There was lower abdominal cramping pain, considerable meteorism and borborygmi especially at night.

She reported loss of appetite and 15 lb unintentional weight loss in approximately 12–18 months. She prefers to eat frequent and small meals, but denies nausea, vomiting, early satiety, or dysphagia.

She had tried polyethylene glycol, multiple fiber supplements and more recently lubiprostone, with no significant improvement in the symptoms.

About 3 years ago she developed suprapubic discomfort with feeling that she has to urinate. She urinates several times a night. But, when she is in the bathroom, she is not always able to pass urine. She has been told she has incomplete bladder emptying.

She also noted difficulty focusing and blurry vision 3 years ago.

About 12–18 months ago she started suffering from syncopal episodes that occurred when she was sitting on the toilet and straining. She had six of them in a short period. Afterwards she started complaining of light-headedness and, at times, of blacking out when standing up from a chair or from a squatting position.

She also complains of no energy, especially on waking up in the morning.

She had a cardiovascular evaluation elsewhere which showed no structural heart disease, a Holter monitor was negative for arrhythmia despite the presence of symptoms; a carotid ultrasound was

33

negative as well. However, she was found to have chronotropic incompetence and orthostatic drop of blood pressure.

She complains of dry mouth, but not dry eyes. Sweating capacity is decreased, resulting in heat intolerance.

Examination

Examination was normal except for presence of Adie's pupils.

Pertinent tests

Complete blood count, electrolytes, neuroimmunology panel, endocrine testing, plasma and urine immunoelectrophoresis, and routine chemistry tests were normal. Fat aspirate was negative for amyloid.

Plasma catecholamines showed supine norepinephrine 37 pg/mL, standing 192 pg/mL. AchR 5.89 nmol/L.

Autonomic study: generalized autonomic failure was present (Figs 9.1–9.4).

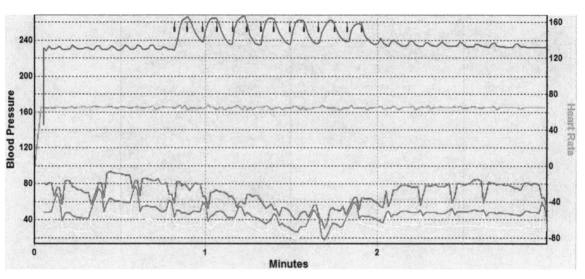

Fig. 9.1 Heart rate response to deep breathing was essentially absent.

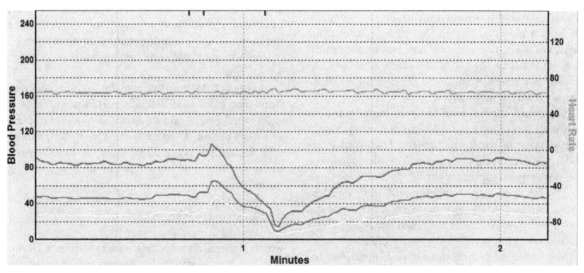

Fig. 9.2 Valsalva maneuver: there is marked reduction of Valsalva ratio, indicating absence of cardiac response, and the blood pressure profile is abnormal, with absence of late phase II and IV and prolonged recovery time.

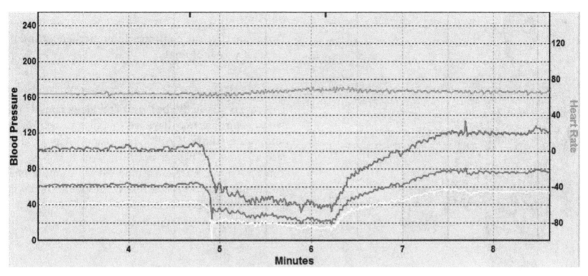

Fig. 9.3 Tilt study showed presence of severe orthostatic hypotension and almost absent cardiac response.

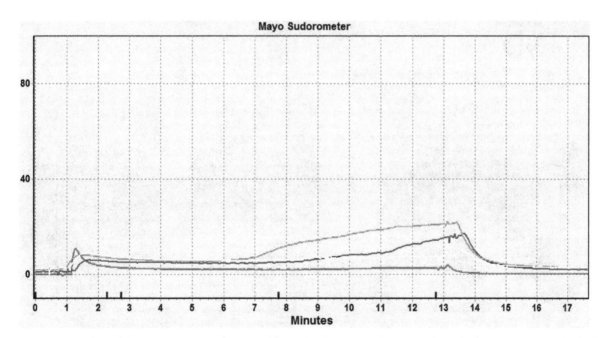

Fig. 9.4 QSART showed absent responses in the forearm and foot, reduced response at the proximal leg and still normal response at the distal leg site.

TST showed 82% anhidrosis (Fig. 9.5).

GI transit: Persistently delayed colonic transit. Mild delayed gastric emptying with normal small bowel transit.

She was started on intravenous immunoglobulin (IVIG), and already at 3 months marked improvement was noted. Repeat autonomic screen showed no change in cardiovagal and cardiosympathetic function, but vasomotor function had improved (Figs 9.6–9.8).

Sudomotor function also showed remarkable recovery on TST (Fig. 9.9).

35

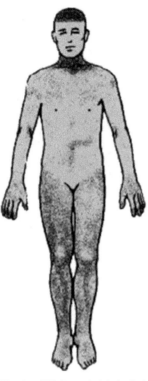

Follow-up

Two years later she continues immunotherapy and is essentially asymptomatic.

Comments

This case is instructive because of the slower onset and progression that may have led to a diagnosis of pure autonomic failure [PAF]. The seropositivity in this case allowed for proper diagnosis, but it is possible some "PAF" cases are more indolent acute autonomic ganglionopathies. Testing for AChR autoantibody is always warranted.

Fig. 9.5 TST showed global anhidrosis, with patchy areas of preserved, albeit light sweat.

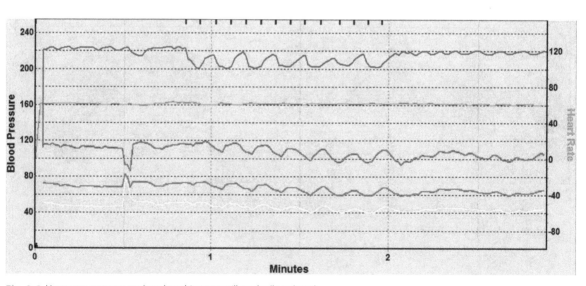

Fig. 9.6 Heart rate response to deep breathing was still markedly reduced.

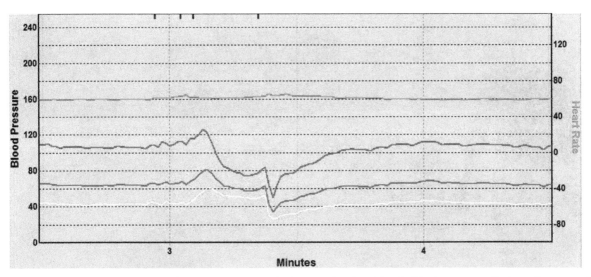

Fig. 9.7 During Valsalva maneuver cardiac responses continued to be severely reduced, but the blood pressure profile showed presence of late phase II and was otherwise unchanged.

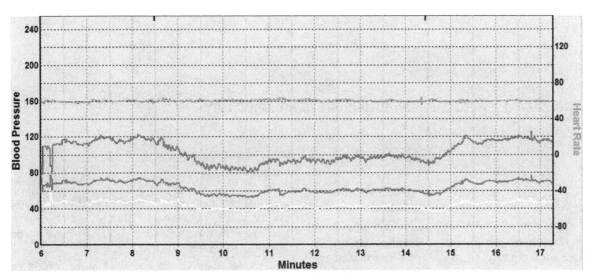

Fig. 9.8 Tilt study: despite the still absent cardiac response, orthostatic blood pressures improved dramatically when compared with the first study, suggesting recovery of peripheral vasoconstriction function (also suggested by the Valsalva profile).

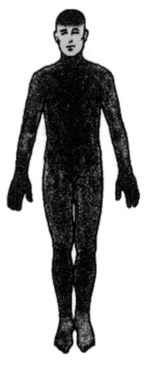

Fig. 9.9 TST showed a normal profile.

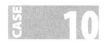 **Autoimmune autonomic ganglionopathy**

History

A 17-year-old male, very athletic, presented 9 months after insidious onset of functional decline. He noticed that he was not recovering well from his workout and at first he thought he was overtraining, so he slowed that down, but that still did not help. He also began to experience postural light-headedness and presyncopal events. He suffered unintentional weight loss, despite the fact he had a more than adequate food intake, by description, and began to develop some constipation. He had no symptoms of dry eyes or dry mouth, and reported no bladder dysfunction. He noticed that he would sweat much less than before whenever he tried to exercise. He also became extremely sensitive to change in temperature partly due to the fact that he had lost 30 lb in about 6 months. When he was evaluated, he was found to have an extremely low heart rate, in the 20s, and a pacemaker was placed which helped to some extent.

Testing done in an outside facility confirmed marked autonomic impairment, including sudomotor failure. His AchR titer was 0.06 nmol/L, which is a very low positive titer. He was started on intravenous immunoglobulin (IVIG) and with some improvement, but it was then stopped due to abnormal liver function studies.

Examination

It showed a thin, pale young man, with an otherwise normal neurologic exam.

Pertinent tests

Hematology, routine chemistry, endocrinology, and neuroimmunology panels were normal except for the AchR titer, which was again positive at low titer of 0.05 nmol/L.

When we repeated the autonomic studies, severe vasomotor and cardiac insufficiency was noted, with mild sudomotor abnormalities (Figs 10.1–10.4) but the TST was normal (Fig. 10.5).

An exercise study revealed reduced exercise tolerance with poor hemodynamic responses.

Norepinephrine levels were 154 and 321 pg/mL supine and standing, respectively (i.e. blunted considering his orthostatic hypotension).

We decided to resume immunotherapy and 9 months later the patient had achieved a complete recovery both clinically and on testing (Figs 10.6–10.9) such that the pacemaker was removed. He has since returned to his athletic career.

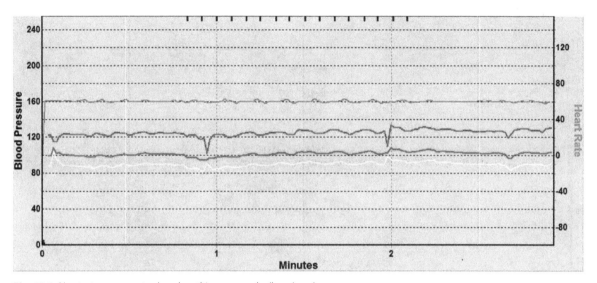

Fig. 10.1 Heart rate response to deep breathing was markedly reduced.

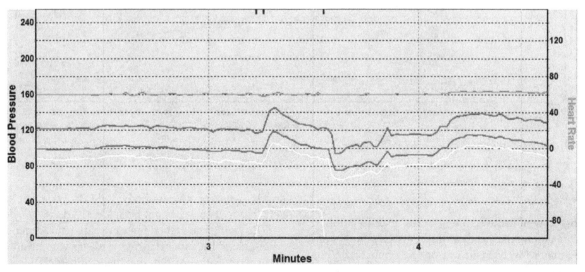

Fig. 10.2 Valsalva maneuver shows severely reduced Valsalva ratio. Blood pressure profile showed a "flat-top" variant, but with markedly prolonged recovery time.

Case 10 Autoimmune autonomic ganglionopathy

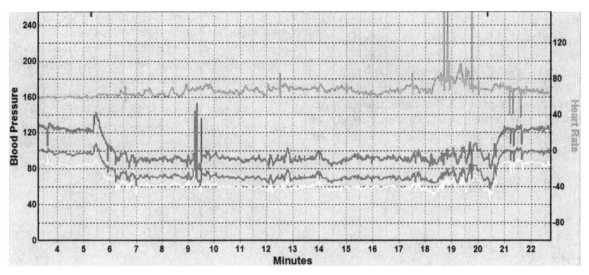

Fig. 10.3 Tilt study showed presence of orthostatic hypotension and severely reduced cardiac response.

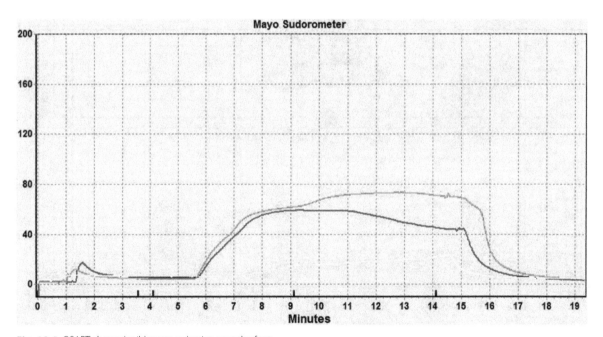

Fig. 10.4 QSART showed mild sweat reduction over the foot.

Comment

This case illustrates the protean manifestation of acute autonomic ganglionopathy [AAG]. In this case the major involvement was on the sympathetic/noradrenergic domain, while cholinergic functions were grossly spared. The low AchR-ab titer would fit that profile. Another autoantibody is likely responsible here, but to date, it has not been identified.

The young age argued for a primary neurodegenerative disorder. An extensive work-up (to exclude particularly genetic and metabolic disorders) was necessary before we could safely conclude this was likely AAG and immunotherapy was warranted.

40

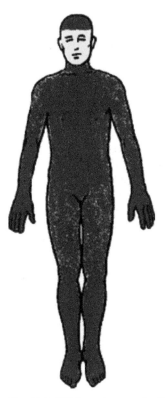

Fig. 10.5 TST showed a normal pattern.

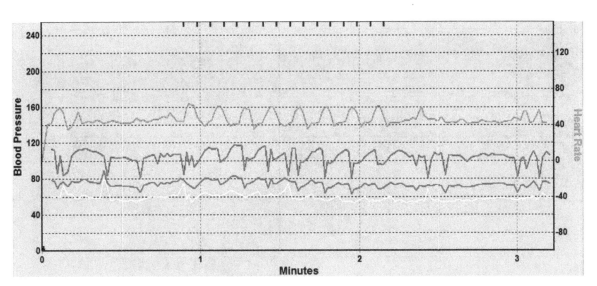

Fig. 10.6 Heart rate response to deep breathing was normal.

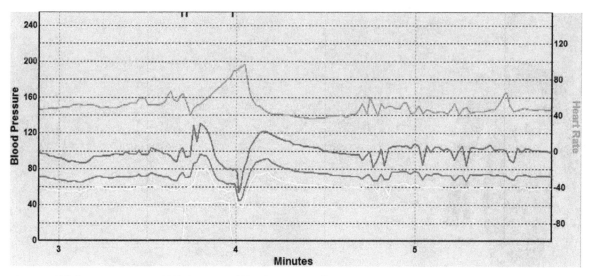

Fig. 10.7 Valsalva maneuver: normal Valsalva ratio and blood pressure profile.

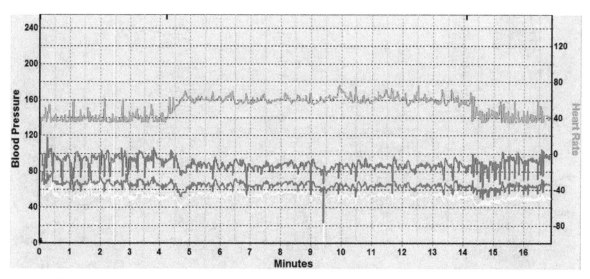

Fig. 10.8 Tilt study: normal.

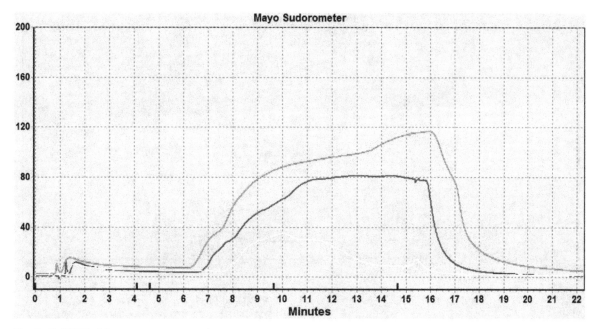

Fig. 10.9 QSART: all the responses are normal.

11 Chronic idiopathic anhidrosis (CIA)

History

A 33-year-old Asian male in general excellent health presented 14 months after one episode of severe light-headedness, palpitations, and becoming overheated while playing tennis. He noticed he was not sweating at that time. Afterwards, he began to realize he was not sweating anymore but, instead, he would feel like scratching and a prickly sensation on his skin in situations when he should be sweating. Also, he noted loss of sweating over palms, soles, and armpits. This had profoundly impacted his ability to exercise outdoors and he had to use external means to cool himself off. He had no other autonomic, neurologic, or systemic symptoms.

Examination

His examination was normal.

Pertinent tests

His blood studies were normal, specifically he had negative AchR serology.

The autonomic screen was normal except for quantitative sudomotor axon reflex test (Fig. 11.1). TST showed global anhidrosis (Fig. 11.2). Skin biopsy showed mild lymphocytic infiltration around sweat glands.

An empiric trial of immunotherapy yielded mild improvement at 3 months (Fig. 11.3) but 3 years later he reported enough sweating capacity over his trunk so that he was able to resume most of his outdoors sport activity without overheating.

Comment

Chronic idiopathic anhidrosis may have an acute or an insidious onset. In some cases we have seen inflammatory infiltrate around sweat glands suggesting immunotherapy may be beneficial. The response to treatment has been variable. This appears to be an isolated syndrome, not evolving into a more generalized autonomic disorder.

Case 11 Chronic idiopathic anhidrosis (CIA)

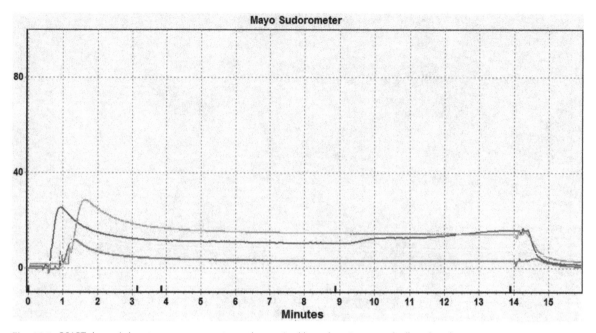

Fig. 11.1 QSART showed absent responses except over the proximal leg, where it was markedly reduced.

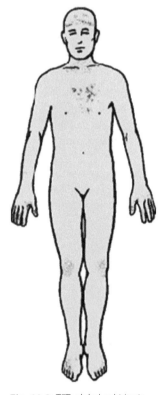

Fig. 11.2 TST: global anhidrosis.

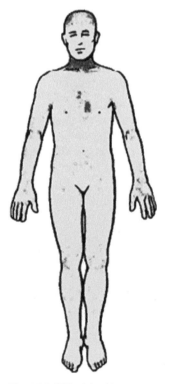

Fig. 11.3 TST: minimal improvement with sweat being present over the neck and small areas of the forehead and chest.

Pseudo chronic idiopathic anhidrosis

History

A 38-year-old male presented for evaluation of recurrent episodes of loss of consciousness. He was extensively evaluated as these spells had mixed features concerning for not only neurocardiogenic syncope, but also partial seizures. Cardiac and epilepsy monitoring were inconclusive but we eventually recognized these events were most likely related to hypoglycemia (as he was diagnosed with diabetes during the evaluations).

As part of his assessment, he underwent a TST. His baseline temperature was normal but it rose very quickly during the study, during which he did not sweat at all (Fig. 12.1). The patient reported no symptoms at the time of the study, but later in the day he informed us he had fallen ill with an upper respiratory infection and had spiked a fever.

We repeated a TST 1 week later, after his illness had resolved and the study was essentially normal (Fig. 12.2).

Comment

The developing illness and fever had altered the patient's sweat threshold, resulting in an abnormal TST. Infections and some medications (such as opiates) alter core temperature and sweat threshold. Thus an abnormal study should be interpreted with caution and ideally repeated once the illness has resolved or medication has been withheld.

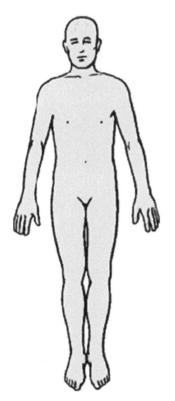

Fig. 12.1 TST: global anhidrosis.

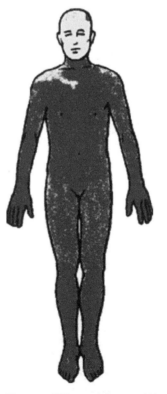

Fig. 12.2 TST: essentially normal (the areas of absent sweat corresponded to prior surgeries and trauma).

History

A 64-year-old male, who has always been healthy, presented for evaluation of progressive loss of sensation in his limbs starting in the feet and then gradually ascending to the arms. Onset began insidiously 5 years prior. During this period of time he also developed erectile dysfunction and diarrhea, which has been diagnosed as irritable bowel syndrome. He has no symptoms suggestive of neurogenic bladder. He has occasional orthostatic light-headedness if he gets up too quickly. He has passed out only once, 2 years ago. He has a history of bradycardia and finally last year he had a pacemaker placed. But no significant changes in his functional status have occurred since. The patient has lost about 50 lb over 5 years, which he attributes to his change in diet because of his diarrhea. He does not report any significant rash or change in skin color, change in body hair, or nails. He has occasional peripheral edema but nothing consistent. He has not injured himself accidentally despite the profound sensory loss and has not fallen despite increasing imbalance. He has noticed weakness particularly in his right hand with occasional fasciculation and a bit of atrophy. He feels overall his symptoms are progressing. He has no cranial nerve impairment except for symptoms of sicca syndrome.

The family history is significant for the fact the patient's grandmother and mother had sensory loss but they were not extensively investigated or diagnosed. He remembers his grandmother being able to take a very hot pan from the stove with her bare hands and not reporting any pain.

Examination

The examination is significant for marked panmodality sensory loss up to the trunk and in a glove distribution, sensory ataxia, mild weakness of the right hand and arm, with mild atrophy. Reflexes are absent.

Pertinent tests

Extensive blood and urine testing (complete blood count, electrolytes, neuroimmunology panel, endocrine testing, plasma and urine immunoelectrophoresis, and routine chemistry tests) were normal except for: platelets = 104×10^9/L, N-terminal probrain natriuretic peptide (NT-proBNP) 3562 (normal < 85 pg/mL).

Electromyography and nerve conduction velocity studies (NCV/EMG) showed the presence of an axonal sensory-motor polyradiculoneuropathy and right median neuropathy at the wrist.

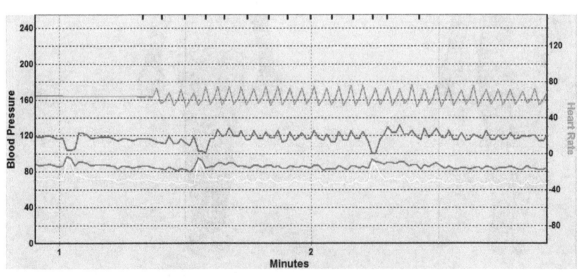

Fig. 13.1(a) Presence of pacemaker and irregular beats makes assessment of heart rate to deep breathing impossible.

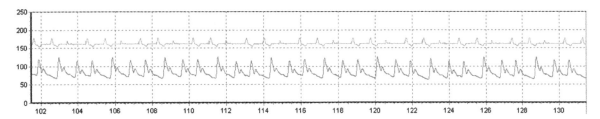

Fig. 13.1(b) ECG strip showing arrhythmia.

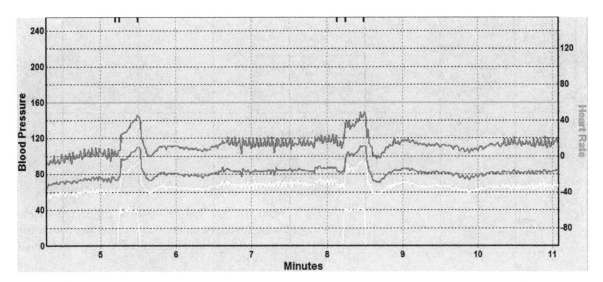

Fig. 13.2 Valsalva maneuver: blood pressure profile shows "flat-top/square wave" morphology that does not change with slight bed tilting (2nd maneuver). Such a pattern is characteristic of heart failure.

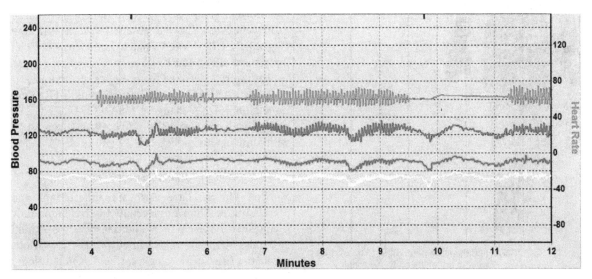

Fig. 13.3 Tilt study shows no significant abnormalities.

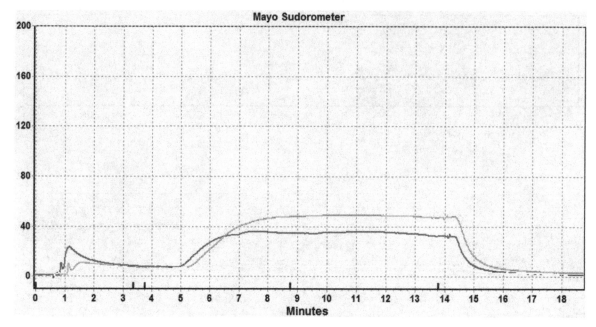

Fig. 13.4 QSART showed normal responses in the leg but markedly reduced response over the foot.

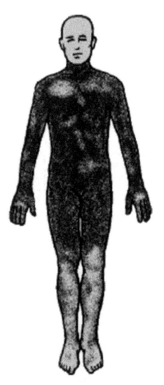

Fig. 13.5 TST: distal anhidrosis was present, with additional patchy areas of reduced sweat over the rest of the body and anhidrosis of the forehead.

Quantitative sensory testing confirmed markedly impaired sensation of all modalities, consistent with a neuropathy affecting both large and small fibers.

Autonomic reflex screen: due to pacemaker, cardiac responses could not be assessed (Fig. 13.1a, b). There was flat-top profile of blood pressure on Valsalva that did not change with slight tilt, suggesting heart failure (Fig. 13.2) but the tilt study was still normal (Fig. 13.3). A quantitative sudomotor axon reflex test showed absent sweat in the foot (Fig. 13.4). TST showed a patchy anhidrosis (22% of body surface; Fig. 13.5).

Fat aspirate detected the presence of amyloid.

Genetic testing identified a pathogenic TTR mutation, Exon: 3; DNA change: c.238A > G (ACT > GCT); amino acid change: p.T60A (Thr60Ala), consistent with familial amyloidosis.

Comments

Amyloidosis can have various manifestations and presentations. Almost universally there is autonomic involvement. Weight loss and sensory loss should also raise suspicion. Cases may present to various specialties (gastroenterology, cardiology, nephrology) based on their most prominent symptoms.

In this case, the presence of a pacemaker prevented assessment of cardiovagal and cardiosympathetic function, but heart rate variability is often lost early in the course of the disease. The presence of a fixed (i.e., not changing with slight bed tilting) flat-top profile in this circumstance suggests congestive heart failure, supported also by the abnormal NT-pro BNP level.

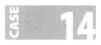

14 Amyloidosis

History

A 46-year-old male presented with a 2–3-year history of increasing gait difficulties. He noticed initial difficulty with running, and then noticed he slapped his feet when walking. He subsequently required a walking aid and at presentation was wheelchair bound. He reported his hands became affected a few months prior to presentation at our institution. During this period of time, he had also begun to experience sensory loss in a stocking distribution. Evaluation in an outside facility revealed elevated cerebrospinal fluid protein and abnormal electromyography. He was diagnosed with chronic inflammatory demyelinating polyneuropathy [CIDP] and started on immunotherapy but he continued to worsen. He lost some weight in the beginning when he had an episode of gastroenteritis but had stabilized since. He had no fever, joint swelling, rash or any systemic symptoms except for fatigue. He reported a progressive difficulty with his sexual function. He also had been bothered by severe constipation and possibly had been having difficulty with emptying his bladder completely. He had no other symptoms of autonomic involvement. He specifically denies any light-headedness and no change in sweat production.

One maternal uncle had died of amyloidosis, but no other family member was reportedly affected.

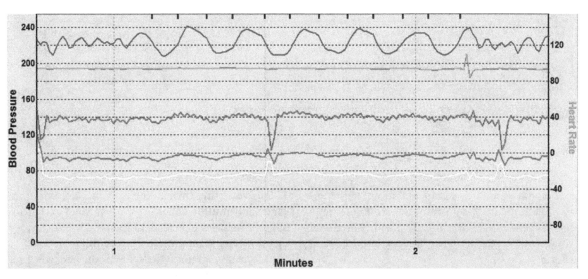

Fig. 14.1 Heart rate response to deep breathing was absent.

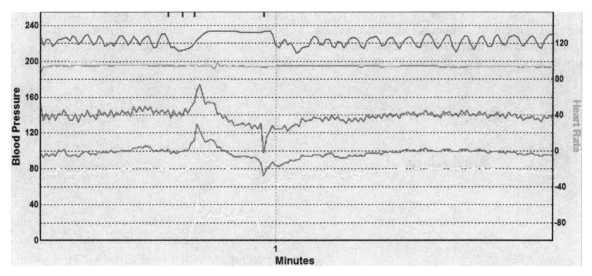

Fig. 14.2 Valsalva maneuver showed complete absence of cardiac responsiveness, while blood pressure profile showed absence of late phase II and IV with prolonged recovery time.

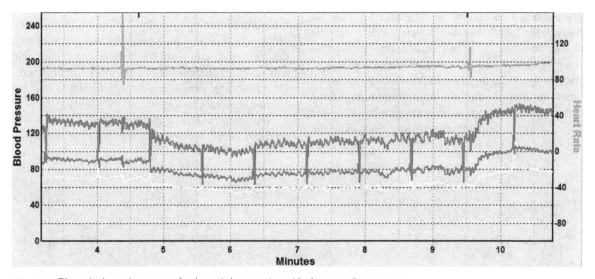

Fig. 14.3 Tilt study showed presence of orthostatic hypotension with absent cardiac response.

Examination

Examination showed a significant motor and sensory involvement, with profound weakness in a length-dependent (but already with proximal involvement) pattern, dense hypo/anesthesia and areflexia.

Pertinent tests

Extensive testing (hematologic, endocrine, immunologic, and routine chemistry) was normal except for slightly reduced platelets (132×10^9/L) and elevated cerebrospinal fluid protein (235mg/dL).

Electromyography NCV/EMG showed the presence of a severe axonal neuropathy.

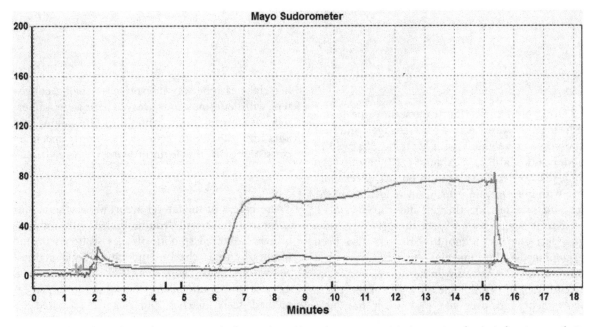

Fig. 14.4 QSART showed normal response over the forearm, but with persistent sweat activity (suggestive of early dysfunction, manifesting as denervation supersensitivity), while in the lower limb the responses were markedly reduced.

Quantitative sensory testing revealed that he was insensitive to all modalities. Autonomic reflex screen showed evidence of marked cardiovagal and adrenergic dysfunction, with distal sudomotor impairment (Figs 14.1–14.4).

An echocardiogram revealed marked increase in wall thickness.

Fat aspirate: it was positive for amyloid.

Nerve biopsy: there was severe loss of all fiber types, with the presence of axonal degeneration and amyloid deposition around blood vessels and in the endoneurial space.

Genetic testing detected a single Met30 mutation in the prealbumin gene consistent with familial amyloidosis.

Comment

This case simply demonstrates another presentation of transthyretin-related amyloidosis, which may look like CIDP at times, when the somatic component precedes the autonomic manifestations. The elevated cerebrospinal fluid protein is present in both, but the neuropathy is axonal, mimicking the axonal variant of CIDP. The lack of response to treatment and the onset of autonomic symptoms should have raised suspicion. CIDP rarely has autonomic dysfunctions and if present, they are generally mild. The autonomic testing profile showed a classic marked loss of heart rate variability in this case.

History

A 27-year-old female from Indonesia came to the USA over 2 years ago. As a teenager she was exposed to a neighbor with leprosy. She was in good health until approximately 18 months ago when she noticed discoloration on her cheeks and nose with burning and pruritus. The lesions on the face and ears became thicker and she developed the loss of her eyebrows approximately 6 months ago. Over the last 6 months she has also been developing discoloration and erythema associated with pruritus and burning on her upper and lower extremities and trunk. She now has widespread involvement and over the past week has been developing more significant numbness and swelling of her feet, greater than hands, associated with fevers and chills. She has not been on any treatments for leprosy. A biopsy obtained from her right earlobe was interpreted as being consistent with lepromatous leprosy. There were numerous organisms seen with the Fite stain and auramine/rhodamine stain in her biopsy specimen consistent with this form of leprosy.

Examination

There is loss of the lateral eyebrows, erythematous indurated thickened leonine facies with reddish-brown indurated smooth plaques scattered on the forehead, nose, cheeks, and chin; erythematous, edematous palms and soles. She had ill-defined, discrete and confluent, erythematous to hyperpigmented scaly patches and plaques scattered on the arms, forearms, thighs, and legs. She had more diffuse erythema with ill-defined, coalescent papules scattered on the back, chest, and abdomen.

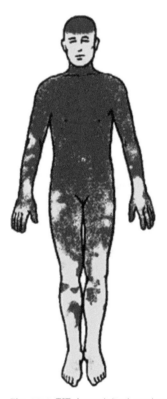

Fig. 15.1 TST showed distal, patchy anhidrosis, corresponding to the affected skin areas.

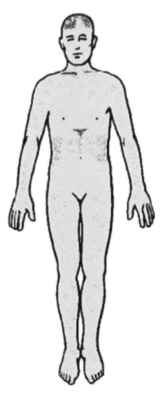

Fig. 15.2 First TST was done when the patient was febrile and showed global anhidrosis (see also case #12).

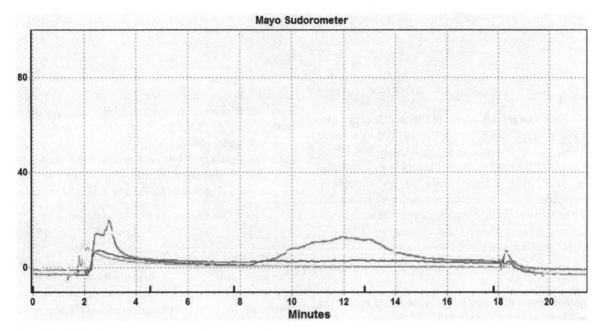

Fig. 15.3 QSART showed absent responses in the lower limb.

Reflexes are normal, but there are marked alterations in sensation which are over the lobules of the ears for pinprick, over the malar surface, over both hands, and to an asymmetric degree in the legs. Subjectively, she describes altered feeling over the distribution of the right superficial peroneal nerve, and over the distal plantar nerves. She has marked loss of vibration in the toes. Joint position is almost normal. Touch pressure is clearly abnormal, and pinprick is especially abnormal over these regions.

Pertinent tests

Routine blood work was unremarkable.

TST: there are patchy, confluent areas of anhidrosis mainly over cooler areas of the body (30% anhidrosis) (Fig. 15.1). (Of note, the first time she was tested she was febrile (Fig. 15.2 – fever) and had global anhidrosis (see also Case 12): the test repeated 3 weeks later showed the pattern described above.)

Autonomic reflex screen: normal, except for distal sudomotor abnormalities (Fig. 15.3).

Quantitative sensory testing: patient was insensitive to all sensory modalities.

NCV/EMG showed the presence of an axonal, length-dependent peripheral neuropathy.

Nerve biopsy: decreased density of myelinated fibers (severe). Increased number of empty nerve strands. Sheets of inflammatory cells and granuloma formation, some disrupting small vessel walls. Rare multi-nucleated giant cells. Extensive infiltration of all nerve components by acid fast bacilli. Onion skin appearance of the perineurium. Diagnostic of leprosy.

Comment

This is a textbook example of this condition, with classic involvement of cooler areas of the body.

Dopamine–beta-hydroxylase deficiency

History

A 15-year-old female presented with a lifelong history of syncope and collapse. The patient had severe orthostatic intolerance and consistently low blood pressure readings. Despite maximal symptomatic treatment, the patient continued to experience severe symptoms. However, she had no other autonomic symptoms that would suggest familial dysautonomia. Her family history was negative for similar problems.

Examination

There was slow pupillary light response, otherwise the examination was unremarkable.

Pertinent tests

The patient's supine and standing epinephrine and norepinephrine levels were less than 10 pg/mL (normal = 70–750 pg/mL). Her dopamine levels were 227 and 301 pg/mL supine and standing, respectively, with normal being < 30, with no postural change.

Autonomic reflex screen: severe noradrenergic failure was present, while cardiovagal and sudomotor functions were preserved, except for absent response on the foot (Figs 16.1–16.4), but TST was normal (Fig. 16.5).

Comments

The clinical history and catecholamine results are pathognomonic for dopamine–beta-hydroxylase deficiency. The condition is exceedingly rare and responds to L-threo-dihydroxyphenylserine (L-DOPS) therapy. L-DOPS converts to norepinephrine, bypassing the step normally performed by the absent enzyme. Such therapy essentially allows the patients to have a normal life, which is what happened to this patient.

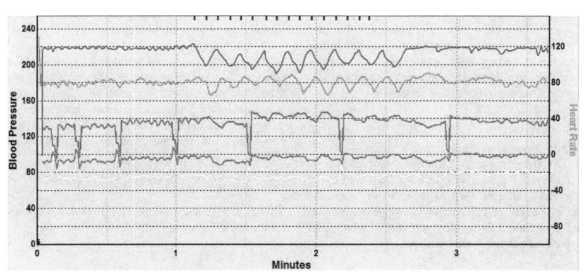

Fig. 16.1 Heart rate response to deep breathing was normal.

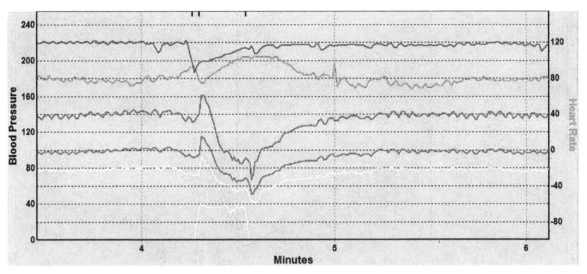

Fig. 16.2 Valsalva maneuver: Valsalva ratio was normal, but the blood pressure profile showed markedly attenuated late phase II, absence of phase IV, and prolonged recovery time.

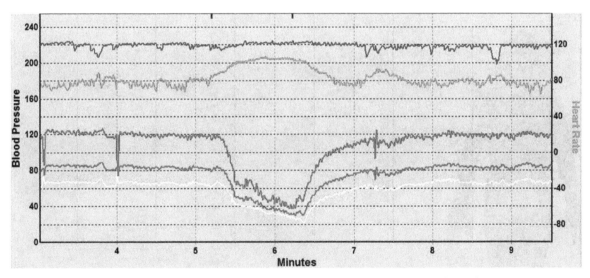

Fig. 16.3 Tilt study detected severe orthostatic hypotension, while a cardiac response was still present but inadequate.

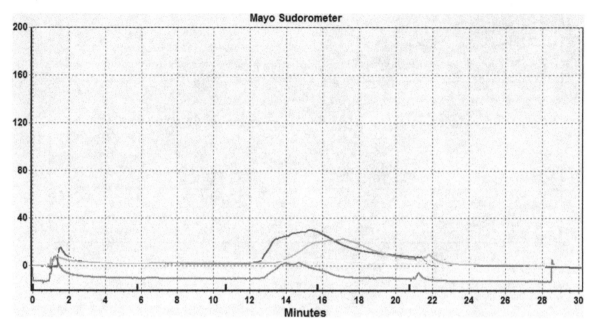

Fig. 16.4 QSART showed absent response in the foot, normal at the other sites.

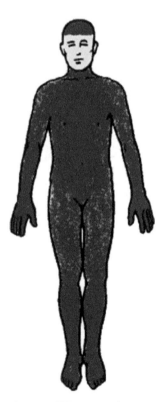

Fig. 16.5 TST was normal.

Hereditary sensory and autonomic neuropathy type I + CIA

History

A 60-year-old male presented with an approximately 10-year history of troublesome heat intolerance. He noted that he would sweat only on the right side of his chest and left leg. With exertion especially on a warm day he would feel weak and light-headed and fatigued. Cooling would alleviate the symptoms. His bowel pattern had been abnormal for approximately 5 years with loose stools two to three times per day and occasional accidental soiling. About 4 years prior to presentation he developed some numbness affecting the right lateral thigh with some radiation down the lateral leg. About 2 years prior to presentation he had developed numbness of his feet. The patient had changes in the skin of his extremities, with dry skin and loss of skin appendages such as hair. He is bothered by pruritus, particularly of his lower extremities and also in his forearms.

At the same time he also began to complain of dry mouth and orthostatic light-headedness, which were particularly troublesome in the morning. He has had significant erectile dysfunction and also has some mild urgency of micturition. Of note is that he has a maternal aunt and a mother who have painful feet and heat intolerance.

He was found to have a small IgG lambda monoclonal gammopathy that has remained unchanged.

Examination

There was glove and stocking distribution panmodality sensory loss with no weakness. He was areflexic in the lower extremities. There were reduced pupillary responses.

Pertinent tests

Laboratory tests: plasma catecholamines were normal. IgG lambda peak was small and stable when compared with prior levels. All other routine (including endocrine and neuroimmunology panel), blood, and urine tests were normal.

NCV/EMG showed evidence of an axonal sensory neuropathy.

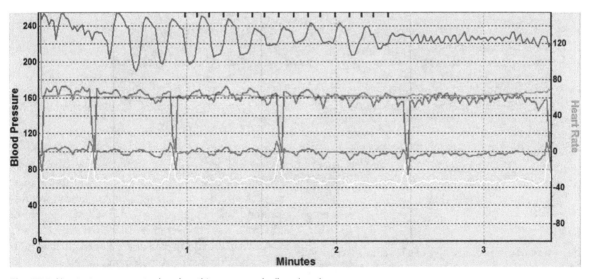

Fig. 17.1 Heart rate responses to deep breathing were markedly reduced.

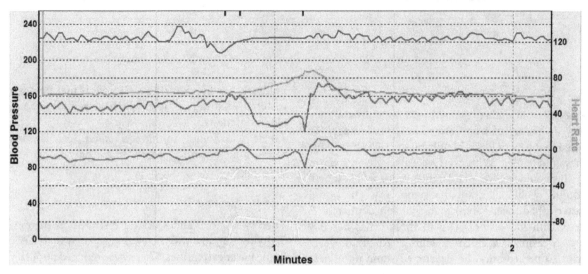

Fig. 17.2 Valsalva maneuver showed a borderline normal Valsalva ratio for age and normal blood pressure profile.

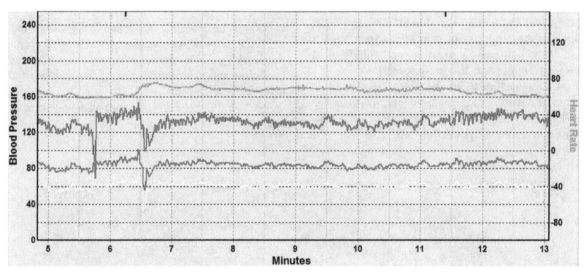

Fig. 17.3 Tilt study showed transient orthostatic hypotension with rapid recovery, suggesting mild vasoconstrictor insufficiency. Such a pattern can also be seen in hypovolemia, deconditioning, and antihypertensive treatment.

Autonomic reflex screen: there were abnormal sudomotor and cardiovagal functions, with transient orthostatic hypotension (Figs 17.1–17.4).

TST: global anhidrosis (Fig. 17.5).

Comment

The history was most suggestive of a hereditary sensory and autonomic neuropathy type 1 [HSAN1] form. The pattern did not fit with a neuropathy associated to monoclonal gammopathy of unknown significance [MGUS] as onset preceded the MGUS appearance, the peak size did not change despite clinical progression, and the neuropathy was axonal. The degree of anhidrosis was however far greater than expected, and we speculated that the patient developed chronic idiopathic anhidrosis superimposed on HSAN1.

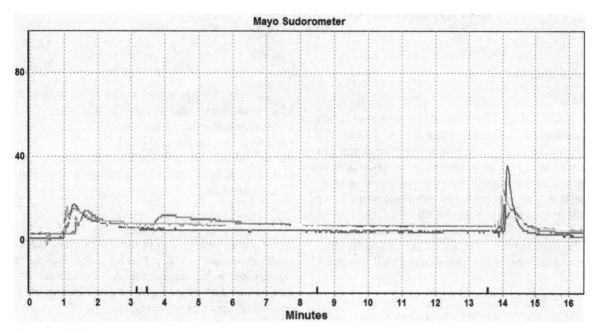

Fig. 17.4 QSART responses were absent for all sites.

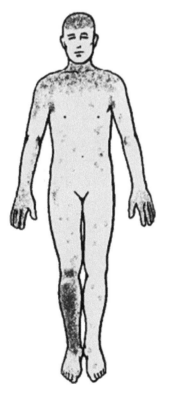

Fig. 17.5 TST showed global anhidrosis with only patchy areas of preserved sweat.

Postural orthostatic tachycardia syndrome with hyperadrenergic storms

History

A 72-year-old female presented with a 30-year history of episodic flushing, hypertension, and palpitations triggered by activity and relieved by lying down. The patient was extensively worked-up for pheochromo-cytoma, carcinoid (although she had more constipation than diarrhea), primary hyperaldosteronism, and mastocytosis with negative results.

She had no other autonomic symptoms.

Repeat testing once again did not detect any abnormality that could explain her clinical syndrome.

Examination

The examination was entirely normal.

Pertinent tests

Hematologic, endocrine, routine chemistry, and neuroimmunology panel were normal.

A 24-hour blood pressure Holter monitor showed labile hypertension and tachycardia (Fig. 18.1).

Autonomic reflex screen showed normal cardio-vagal function, exaggerated blood pressure overshoot during phase IV of Valsalva maneuver, and excessive tachycardia and hypertension on tilt (Figs 18.2–18.4).

Comment

This is an unusual case of postural orthostatic tachy-cardia syndrome [POTS]. POTS is very unusual in this age group, but her symptoms started in her 40s. The paradoxical BP and HR behavior during tilt is consistent with a hyperadrenergic state. This variant may be due to central dysregulation, which is likely responsible for the autonomic storms occasionally seen in POTS.

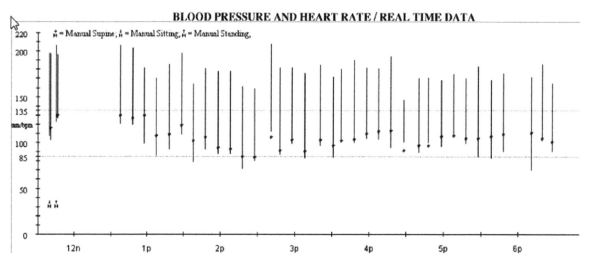

Fig. 18.1 Holter recording showed labile blood pressure and excessive tachycardia.

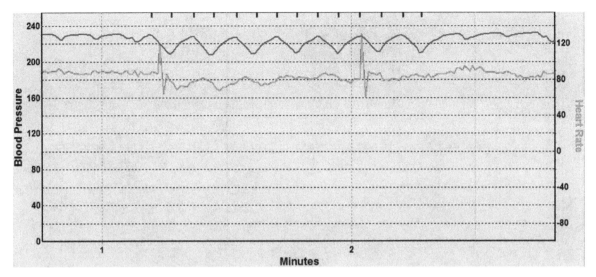

Fig. 18.2 Heart rate response to deep breathing was normal for age.

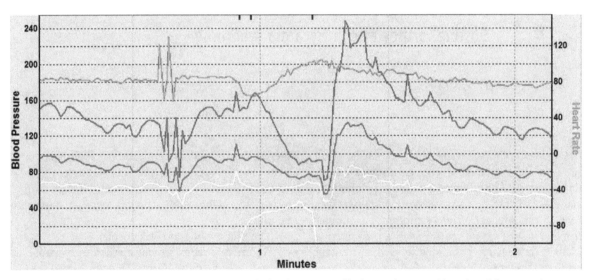

Fig. 18.3 Valsalva maneuver: cardiac responses are normal. Blood pressure profile shows a low normal late phase II for age and an exaggerated phase IV overshoot.

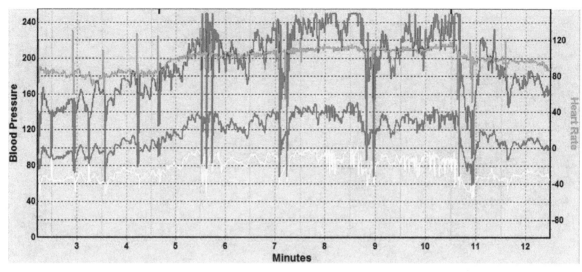

Fig. 18.4 Tilt study showed hypertensive response and inappropriate tachycardia.

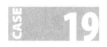

Postural orthostatic tachycardia syndrome

History

A 36-year-old female began to have problems at the age of 18 years after she developed a severe case of mononucleosis. She began to experience palpitations, sweating, irritable bowel syndrome, and was diagnosed with anxiety. Her symptoms continued throughout subsequent years, and she continued to feel light-headed upon standing as well as noticing excessive palpitations. She had a few syncopal events, but she generally has enough warning to sit down and protect herself. She cannot exercise much because of her very poor stamina. She has no other autonomic symptoms except for the irritable bowel, which is diarrhea predominant. She has a history of migraines, which have been fairly well controlled. She reports her sleep quality is quite good, but still she is exhausted at the end of the working day and oftentimes needs a nap before dinner.

Examination

The examination was normal.

Pertinent tests

Hematologic, endocrine, routine chemistry, and neuroimmunology panel were normal except for low vitamin D levels. Plasma catecholamines were normal as were the 24-hour urinary sodium output and urine volume.

The echocardiogram was normal.

Autonomic reflex screen: marked tachycardia on tilt, but was otherwise normal (Figs 19.1–19.4).

TST: normal.

Exercise study: normal hemodynamic profile but profound deconditioning (VO_2 max = 61% of that predicted for age).

Comment

This is a classic case of postural orthostatic tachycardia syndrome [POTS]. Acute onset after mononucleosis is relatively common. Also common is the constellation of fatigue, migraine, and irritable bowel syndrome associated with the orthostatic intolerance, indicating a more pervasive dysfunction and autonomic

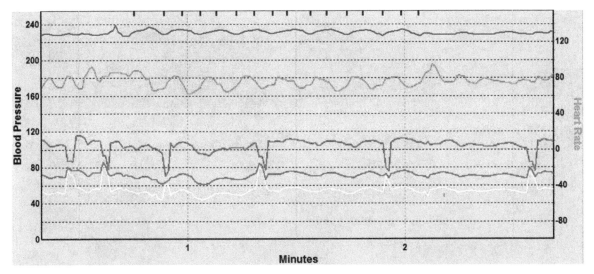

Fig. 19.1 Heart rate responses to deep breathing were normal.

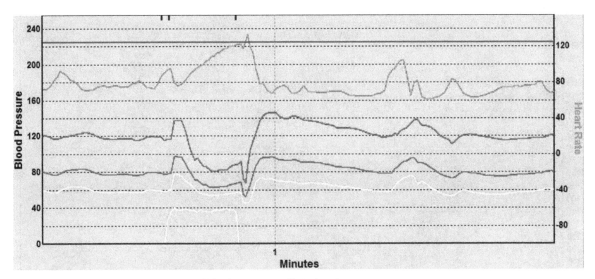

Fig. 19.2 Valsalva maneuver showed normal blood pressure profile and cardiac responses.

instability. Other common complaints include interstitial cystitis, cognitive difficulties, sleep difficulties, diffuse pain (fibromyalgia-like), and dysthymia.

Management should thus address the whole cluster, not just the orthostatic intolerance, for a successful outcome.

Profound deconditioning, hypovolemia, excessive venous pooling in the lower limb, chronic fatigue, and severe anxiety may all present with similar features. Thus such diagnosis should not be overused or misused.

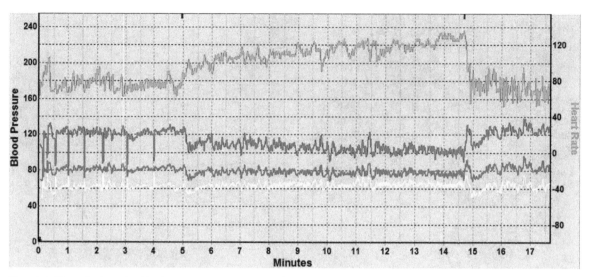

Fig. 19.3 Tilt study showed mild pulse pressure compression and exaggerated tachycardic response.

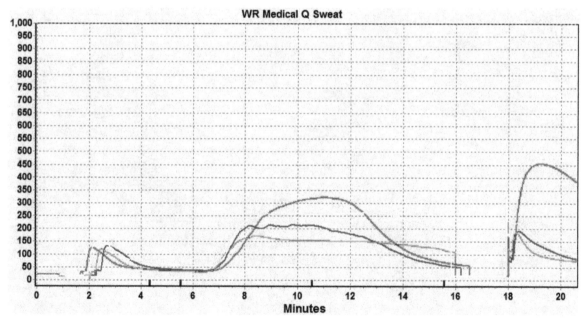

Fig. 19.4 QSART was normal at all sites.

History

A 63-year-old male presented for management of extremely labile blood pressure. His history was quite unusual and complex. He had undergone two suboccipital craniectomies to control unrelenting coughing spells that started after two rear-end road traffic accidents. The first surgery was successful in relieving his symptoms and caused no problems. Unfortunately after the second one (the details of which were unclear) he began to experience large blood pressure fluctuations, with highs > 220/140 mmHg and lows < 60 mmHg systolic.

He had no other autonomic symptoms. He was very symptomatic during both the high and low episodes, with headaches and transient neurologic deficits. He noticed he had some very specific triggers for these events (such as meals, exertion, etc.) but at other times the events were unprovoked.

Examination

The examination revealed the presence of mild hypernasality in his speech, he had anisocoria with the left pupil being larger but reactive, reflexes were depressed throughout and he had a sensory loss level at T1 to temperature and pinprick.

Pertinent tests

Complete blood count, electrolytes, neuroimmunology panel, endocrine testing, plasma and urine immuno-electrophoresis, and routine chemistry tests were normal. Plasma norepinephrine was 477 and 314 pg/mL supine and standing, respectively (opposite of that expected).

The autonomic reflex screen detected the presence of adrenergic and cardiovagal dysfunction while postganglionic sudomotor function was intact (Figs 20.1–20.4).

The TST was normal (Fig. 20.5).

Brain MRI/MRA were normal except for postsurgical changes, but no other abnormality was seen.

MRI of the spine was normal.

BP/HR Holter monitoring: marked fluctuations in BP >> HR (Fig. 20.6)

A repeat tilt study on medication showed there was still fluctuation in blood pressure but overall improved orthostatic tolerance (Fig. 20.7).

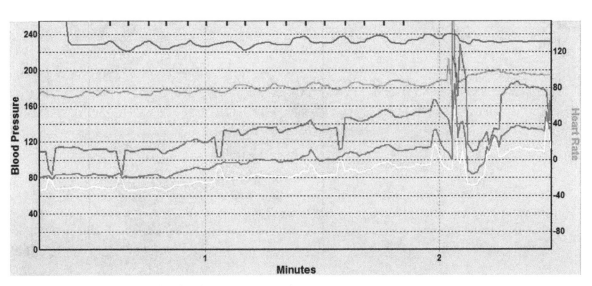

Fig. 20.1 Heart rate responses to deep breathing were attenuated.

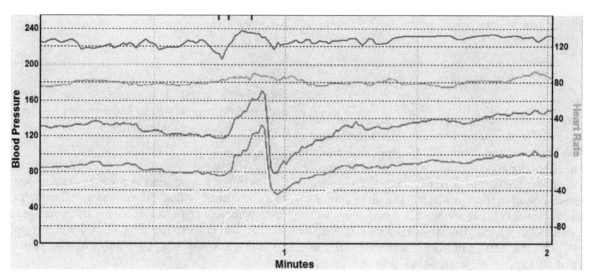

Fig. 20.2 Valsalva maneuver showed marked reduction in cardiac responses, a "flat-top" blood pressure profile with prolonged recovery time, and absent phase IV.

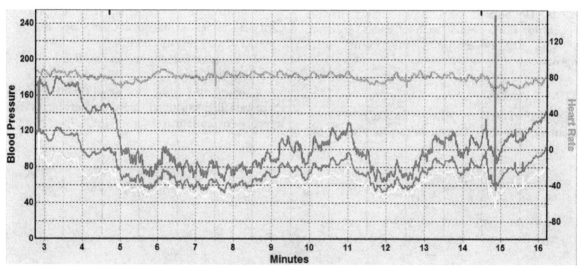

Fig. 20.3 Tilt study showed presence of orthostatic hypotension and absent cardiac response. Note the labile blood pressure throughout the study.

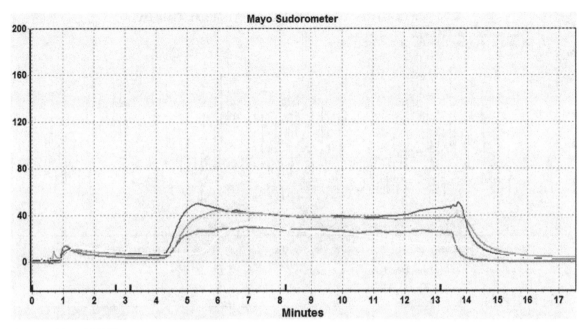

Fig. 20.4 Normal QSART responses.

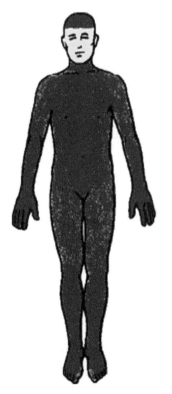

Fig. 20.5 TST was normal.

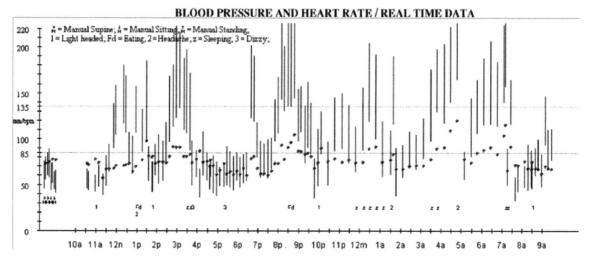

Fig. 20.6 Holter showed extremely labile blood pressure and heart rate.

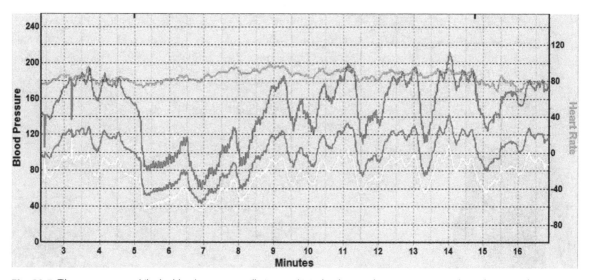

Fig. 20.7 Tilt on treatment: while the blood pressure oscillations and initial orthostatic hypotension persist, his orthostatic tolerance was much improved.

Comment

This case illustrates an extreme example of central dysregulation. His overall hemodynamic profile indicated an exaggerated response to normal stimuli as well as spontaneous oscillations.

His management was complex, requiring expansion of intravascular volume, use of short-acting medications for extreme hyper- and hypotensive readings (often timed to specific triggers such as meals), centrally acting agents (i.e. clonidine) to partially control the amplitude of blood pressure oscillations combined with standard measures to control orthostatic hypotension.

This is undoubtedly one of the most challenging cases we have faced.

History

A 50-year-old male presented for evaluation of worsening fatigue and dizziness. His history was complex. At the age of 18 years he suffered an episode of Guillain-Barré syndrome, from which he recovered fully. At the age of 19 years he was diagnosed with Hodgkin's lymphoma for which he received radiation to neck and chest. At the age of 26 years he suffered a relapse associated with paraneoplastic neuropathy. He was successfully treated with chemotherapy and did well for over 20 years. Then he gradually began to experience increasing fatigue, dizziness, and presyncopal episodes. He also had a history of hypertension, well controlled on medications.

No other autonomic or neurologic symptom was reported.

Examination

The examination revealed mild muscle atrophy and weakness over the shoulders, corresponding to prior radiation treatment area, but no signs of neuropathy were detectable.

Pertinent tests: routine blood tests, including hematologic, endocrine, and neuroimmunologic studies were normal.

Autonomic reflex screen showed the presence of borderline cardiovagal function, impaired adrenergic responses, and orthostatic hypotension (Figs 21.1–21.4).

The echocardiogram was essential normal, but Holter monitoring showed labile blood pressure (Fig. 21.5).

Pulmonary function test: mild non-specific abnormalities (due to prior radiation therapy).

TST: reduced sweating over neck/shoulders due to prior radiation therapy (Fig. 21.6).

He required medication for high as well as low blood pressure. A repeat Holter monitoring (Fig. 21.7) showed moderate improvement. Physical retraining and lifestyle adjustment to reduce the impact of stress and learn how to pace himself was key to a good functional outcome.

Comments

This case illustrates the long-term effect of radiation therapy on baroreceptors. Overall this man was less affected than other similar patients and certainly much less than Case 18 (who is also much more compromised due to the higher level of site of dysfunction, being essentially an

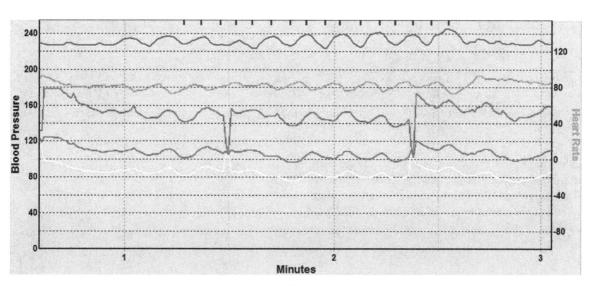

Fig. 21.1 Heart rate responses to deep breathing were borderline for age.

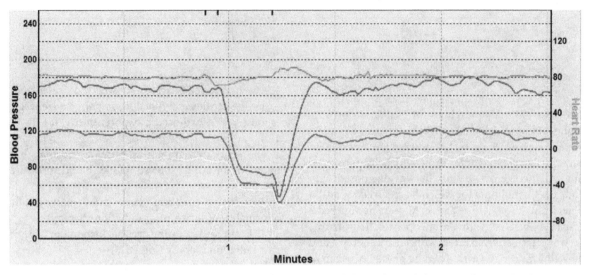

Fig. 21.2 Valsalva maneuver showed marked reduction in cardiac responses, which together with the essentially normal cardiovagal responses points to baroreflex failure. Blood pressure profile showed absence of late phase II and mild prolongation of recovery time.

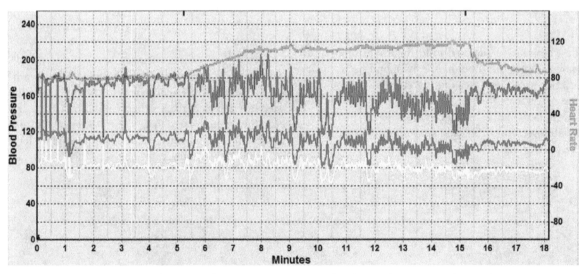

Fig. 21.3 Tilt study showed a gradual decline in blood pressure with end study orthostatic hypotension. Also noted was supine hypertension and labile blood pressure particularly during tilt.

autonomic dysreflexia), but is a good example of the therapeutic challenges these patients represent. With improved survival of cancer patients after radiation, the number of such cases is likely to increase.

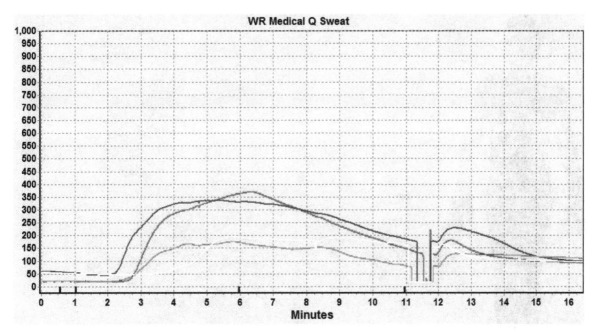

Fig. 21.4 QSART was normal.

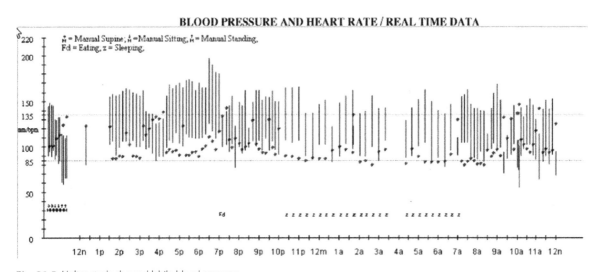

Fig. 21.5 Holter study showed labile blood pressure.

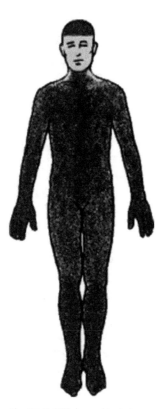

Fig. 21.6 TST showed just absence of sweat in the area of prior radiation therapy.

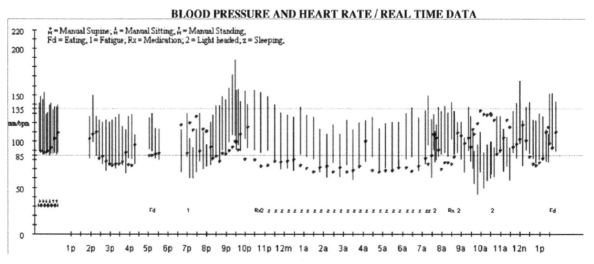

Fig. 21.7 A repeated Holter showed modest improvement on therapy.

History

A 24-year-old female with a history of poorly controlled diabetes since the age of 18 months presented with a few months' history of diffuse, burning dysesthesias. The onset appeared to follow a significant effort in improving the control of her diabetes, which was successful but she experienced multiple hypoglycemic events. At the same time when the pain started she developed macular edema, sensory loss in her distal limbs, symptoms of gastroparesis, diarrhea, difficulty emptying her bladder fully, and orthostatic light-headedness. Her functional capacity and quality of life had been profoundly affected by this symptom complex.

At the time she came to our attention, she had failed multiple attempts to manage her somatic and visceral symptoms.

Examination

On neurologic examination she had diffusely depressed reflexes, which were absent at the ankles, and stocking distribution sensory loss to small fiber modalities.

Pertinent tests

Her HbA1C had been over 11% for many years, but was 6.6% at presentation. Her extensive laboratory tests were normal except for GAD 65 antibody = 0.11 nmol/L (normal < 0.02) and borderline elevated cerebrospinal fluid protein.

A gastrointestinal transit study confirmed the presence of gastroparesis and urodynamic testing showed presence of mild reduction in bladder contractility with increased post-void residual.

NCV/EMG revealed the presence of sensorimotor peripheral neuropathy with mixed demyelinating and axonal features. Quantitative sensory testing showed pan-modality abnormalities, consistent with a neuropathy that affected both large and small fibers.

Autonomic study showed evidence of generalized autonomic failure (Figs 22.1–22.4) and TST (Fig. 22.5) showed a glove-and-stocking distribution of anhidrosis, consistent with involvement of autonomic fibers in the patient's neuropathy.

The patient was started on intravenous methylprednisolone while adjustments were made to her symptomatic therapy for pain, orthostatic

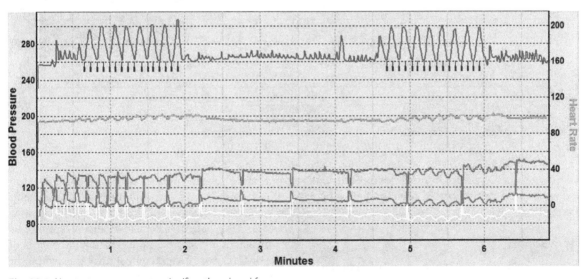

Fig. 22.1 Heart rate responses were significantly reduced for age.

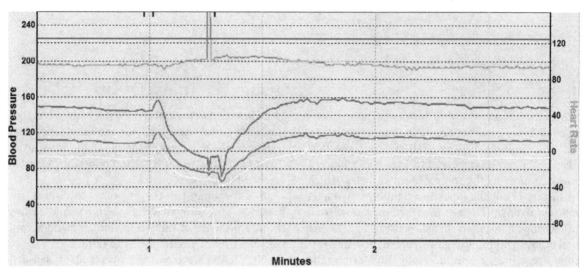

Fig. 22.2 Valsalva maneuver: there was marked impairment of cardiac responses. Blood pressure profile showed absence of late phase II, prolonged recovery time, and markedly reduced phase IV.

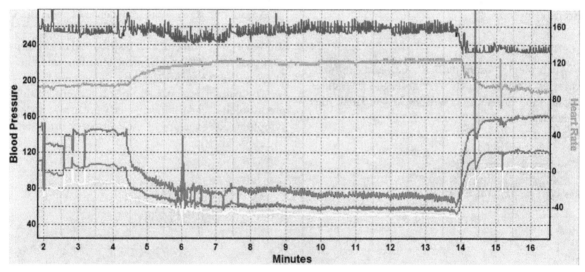

Fig. 22.3 Tilt study showed presence of severe orthostatic hypotension with inadequate compensatory tachycardia.

hypotension, and gastrointestinal dysmotility. A gradual improvement occurred over the following 3 months.

Comments

This case is an example of the extent of neurologic manifestations that can occur with a too drastic and rapid glucose correction in patients with a long-standing history of poorly controlled diabetes. Most commonly patients present with severe, diffuse dysesthesia (also known as insulin neuritis or treatment-induced neuropathy), which is likely due to cytokine release. This patient also had dramatic autonomic involvement at the same time. Treatment consists of a less aggressive glucose control until the symptoms resolve. Immunotherapy can be considered to reduce cytokine levels and reduce inflammation, combined with symptomatic management.

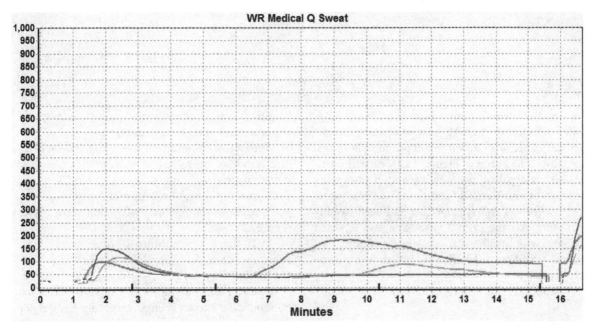

Fig. 22.4 QSART showed normal forearm response but reduced (distal leg) or absent (proximal leg and foot) responses in the lower limb.

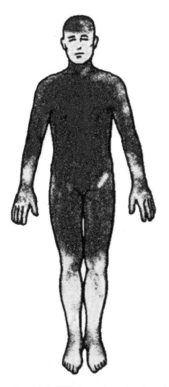

Fig. 22.5 TST showed predominantly distal anhidrosis.

History

A 44-year-old female with a history of poorly controlled diabetes type I for 18 years presented for management of her diabetes with multiple complications. Her HbA1C had been as high as 14.5. She had documented retinopathy, neuropathy, and nephropathy for several years. Her chief complaint was orthostatic light-headedness and syncope that had been steadily worsening over the prior 3 years. She also reported problems with constipation, occasional vomiting (but no clear symptoms suggesting the presence of gastroparesis), and reduced sweating but denied any bladder dysfunction, xerophthalmia, or xerostomia.

Examination

Her neurologic examination revealed a dense stocking distribution pan-modality sensory loss, with depressed deep tendon reflexes, but was otherwise normal.

Blood tests

Selected blood tests included: Hb = 10.3, creatinine = 1.5, eGFR = 38 (normal > 60), HbA1C = 13.3, NT-ProBNP = 1004 (normal < 140 pg/mL), troponin T = 0.14 (normal < 0.01 ng/mL).

Pertinent tests

Cardiac evaluation revealed only non-specific abnormalities of no clinical concern.

Autonomic reflex screen: severe impairment of cardiac responses consistent with diabetic cardiac autonomic neuropathy, impaired vasomotor responses with orthostatic hypotension, and length-dependent postganglionic sudomotor dysfunction were present (Figs 23.1–23.4).

TST: there was anhidrosis over the feet and over an area of the left thorax (T8 level; Fig. 23.5).

One year later the studies were repeated: there were no significant interim changes except for the development of marked supine hypertension and tachycardia (Figs 23.6–23.8).

Comment

This is a fairly classic example of advanced diabetic autonomic neuropathy. The only unusual aspect here was the absence of significant gastrointestinal involvement. Cardiac involvement and diabetic nephropathy are key, independent predictors of poor prognosis. Gastroparesis, constipation, neurogenic bladder, and loss of sweating

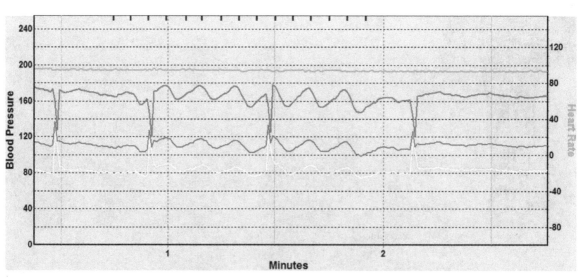

Fig. 23.1 Heart rate response to deep breathing was absent.

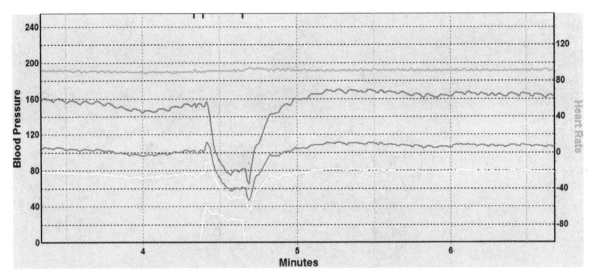

Fig. 23.2 Valsalva maneuver: cardiac responses are almost absent. Blood pressure profile showed attenuation of late phase II and IV with prolonged recovery time.

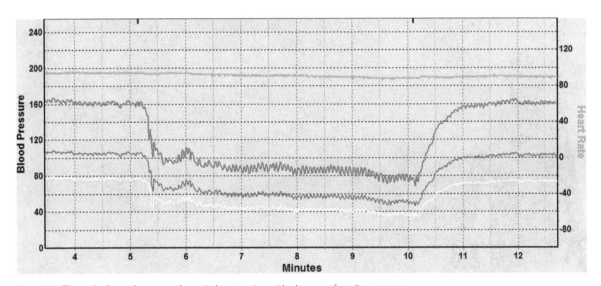

Fig. 23.3 Tilt study showed severe orthostatic hypotension with absence of cardiac response.

with compensatory hyperhidrosis, usually in the cranoiocervical region, profoundly impact quality of life and are often present in this patient population.

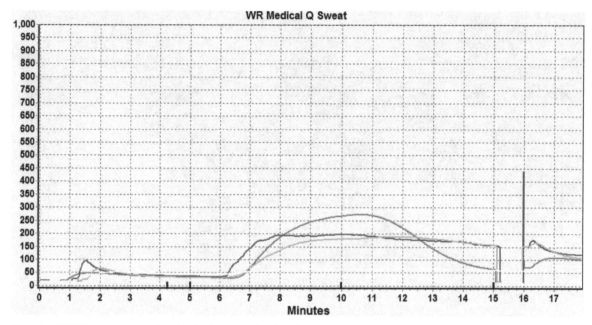

Fig. 23.4 QSART response was reduced in the foot, normal at the other sites.

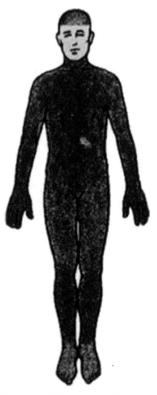

Fig. 23.5 TST showed reduced sweat over the feet, an area of the left chest and the forehead.

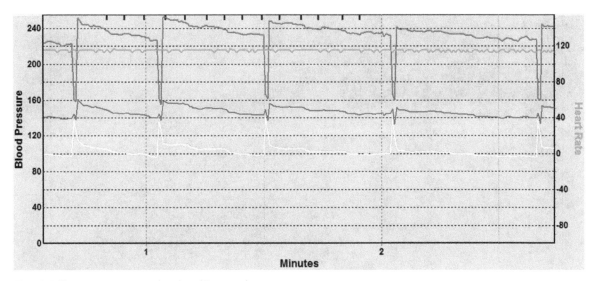

Fig. 23.6 Heart rate response to deep breathing was absent.

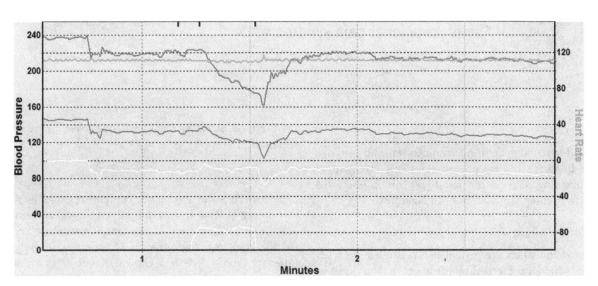

Fig. 23.7 Valsalva maneuver: cardiac responses are absent. Blood pressure profile showed absence of late phase II and IV with prolonged recovery time.

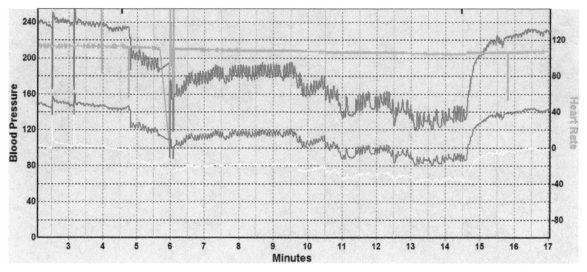

Fig. 23.8 Tilt study showed severe orthostatic hypotension with absence of cardiac response. Note the presence of supine hypertension and invariable tachycardia throughout the study.

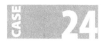

Complex regional pain syndrome

History

A 38-year-old male with chronic lower limb pain due to Buerger's disease presented for management of worsening pain in the left lower limb, associated with swelling, discoloration, and coldness.

Examination

On examination the patient had a swollen, cold left leg, which was mottled bluish in color. The skin was dry and hyperesthetic.

Pertinent tests

On autonomic testing, there was marked vasomotor and sudomotor asymmetry, with cooler temperatures and reduced sweating (Figs 24.1–24.2) over the painful limb.

Comments

The pattern is not specific for complex regional pain syndrome [CRPS] but in the proper clinical context can be very informative. In this case, it was secondary to the long-standing ischemia of the most severely affected limb. CRPS is a clinical diagnosis and the tests can be supportive or suggestive, but cannot rule in or out the diagnosis. Temperature asymmetry may be simply due to disuse, and autonomic instability is common in any neuropathy affecting small fibers, as well as peripheral vascular disease or infections (cellulitis).

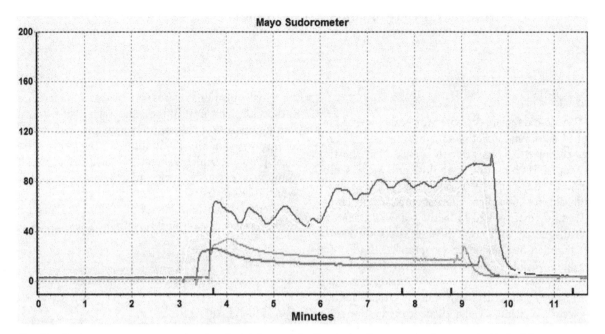

Fig. 24.1 Resting sweat output was reduced on the left foot and distal leg (red and green tracings) compared with the right.

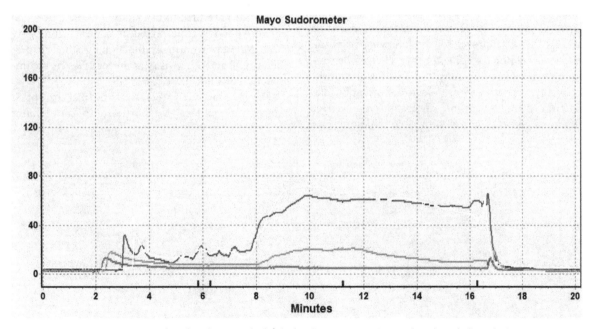

Fig. 24.2 QSART responses were reduced or absent on the left (red and green tracings), normal on the right lower limb.

Pseudo-autoimmune autonomic ganglionopathy (median arcuate ligament syndrome)

History

A 42-year-old female presented for evaluation of presumed autoimmune autonomic disorder. Her history was complex: 5 years prior to presentation she had developed Hashimoto's thyroiditis and sicca symptoms. At the time she began to experience severe stomach and abdominal pain. She underwent cholecystectomy that seemed to help. Meanwhile, she was also diagnosed with celiac disease and started on a strict gluten-free diet. Her symptoms subsided for a while, but then the severe gastrointestinal pain returned, clearly triggered by food intake, associated with nausea and sometimes vomiting. Despite following a strict diet and use of antiemetic medications, her symptom worsened to the point she was unable to maintain adequate oral and food intake. The diagnosis of gastroparesis was made and she required total parenteral nutrition (TPN) for a while, while Botox was given to relax the pylorus, with partial benefit. A pyloroplasty followed and again for a while she appeared to improve. For the following years she periodically required feeding tubes or TPN, while continuing extensive evaluations to define her diagnosis. Eventually, despite lack of serologic confirmation, she was empirically started on hydroxychloroquine. Her symptoms persisted and due to deconditioning and marginal nutritional status she began to experience orthostatic light-headedness. Her review of systems was significant for diffuse body pain that had started during one of her hospitalizations for her gastrointestinal problem, and unilateral loss of hearing, which prompted evaluation for mitochondrial disorder, which was negative.

Her family history was significant for Parkinson's disease, celiac disease, and Hashimoto's thyroiditis.

Examination

Her neurologic examination was entirely normal.

Pertinent tests

Tests included: norepinephrine 325 pg/mL supine and 768 pg/mL standing, mildly positive antinuclear antibody, and abnormalities in blood count due to a recent infection.

A gastrointestinal transit study showed accelerated gastric emptying (interpreted as a post-pyloroplasty effect done on a normally functioning stomach preoperatively) and otherwise was normal. Gastric accommodation was normal.

Her autonomic screen was normal except it showed a pattern of orthostatic intolerance

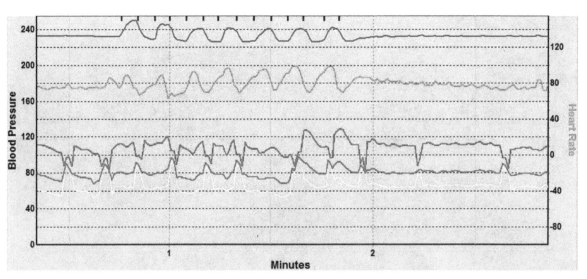

Fig. 25.1 Heart rate responses to deep breathing were normal.

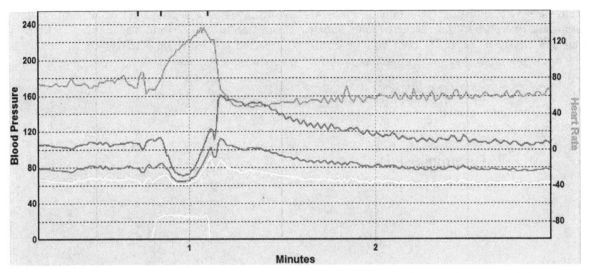

Fig. 25.2 Valsalva maneuver showed normal cardiac responses and normal blood pressure profile except for a prolonged phase IV, suggestive of an hyperadrenergic state.

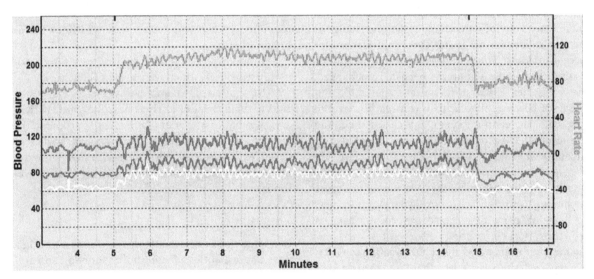

Fig. 25.3 Tilt study showed excessive tachycardia and blood pressure compression, suggesting hypovolemia was responsible for the hyperadrenergic state.

suggestive of relative hypovolemia (Figs 25.1–25.3). Her postganglionic sudomotor and TST were normal (not shown).

Abdominal vessel ultrasound revealed celiac artery stenosis due to arcuate ligament compression.

The patient eventually underwent surgical release with complete resolution of her entire symptomatology.

Comment

This case was obviously complex and many red herrings were present. Nonetheless, the clear correlation between oral intake and onset of symptoms should have triggered the search much sooner. Although autoimmune autonomic ganglionopathy

83

could have very similar presentation, the lack of orthostatic symptoms (that occurred only much later and clearly secondary to poor volume status and deconditioning) and such prominent, painful gastrointestinal symptoms persistent even on duodenal feeding tube, would be unusual. Although suspected clinically, slow transit or gastroparesis were never documented.

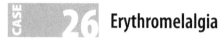

CASE 26 Erythromelalgia

History

A 62-year-old female presented with a 1-year history of periodic flushing and feeling hot in the face and hands. A few months later her lower limbs became involved, with swelling, red discoloration, a very hot sensation in her feet, and intense burning discomfort. There was no obvious preceding trigger, no change in her medications, or her health that could account for these symptoms. There were no systemic symptoms associated, and the symptoms persisted unchanged. She rates her discomfort on average 2/10, but when she becomes hot the pain can reach a level of 8 or 9/10. She cannot tolerate any closed shoe, and whenever she becomes warm, she is extremely uncomfortable, and also her hands and face are involved to a lesser degree. She has no real allodynia, but she keeps her feet out of the covers mainly because her limbs gets warmer when covered and that triggers the burning pain. She denied any focal weakness or sensory loss. Autonomic review of system was negative, but when asked about her sweating capacity, she reported she sweats less than she used to, but attributed it to the fact she had moved to a drier climate area.

Examination

On exam, her legs were slightly edematous and red (Figs 26.1–26.2) but not hot to touch. Subtle sensory loss was present.

Pertinent tests

Routine blood tests, including hematologic, endocrine, and neuroimmunologic studies, were normal.

Quantitative sensory testing: slightly elevated vibratory sensation threshold, but normal thresholds to cold and heat pain, without clear hyperesthesia.

Autonomic reflex screen: normal except for sudomotor responses, which were absent (Fig. 26.3).

TST showed global anhidrosis (Fig. 26.4).

Vascular studies: normal baseline, with patient asymptomatic. As per erythromelalgia protocol, the patient was asked to return during a flare and compared with baseline there were elevated temperatures and laser Doppler flow in the distal lower limbs.

Comment

In a large series, most patients with erythromelalgia have abnormalities of sudomotor function to varying degree, while vasomotor and cardiovagal functions are normal or show only minimal, clinically insignificant, abnormalities. A TST can show involvement of the affected areas, or more widespread dysfunction. Some cases may have a completely normal TST. This syndrome can be secondary (particularly to hematologic disorders), primary/idiopathic, or familial. Cold reproducibly gives

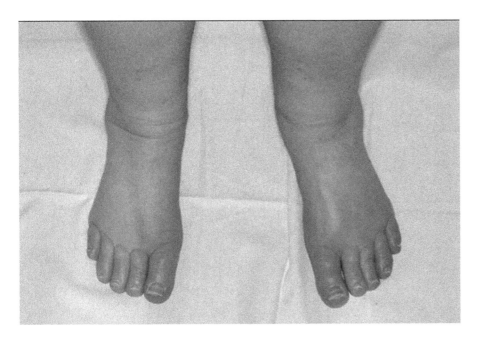

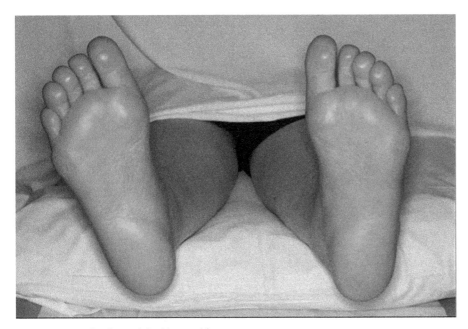

Figs 26.1–26.2 Swollen, red distal legs and feet.

these patients relief. Management includes various topicals and medications commonly used for treatment of neuropathic pain. In acute-onset forms (such as in postviral or postsurgical cases), an autoimmune etiology is the likely culprit and patients respond to immunotherapy.

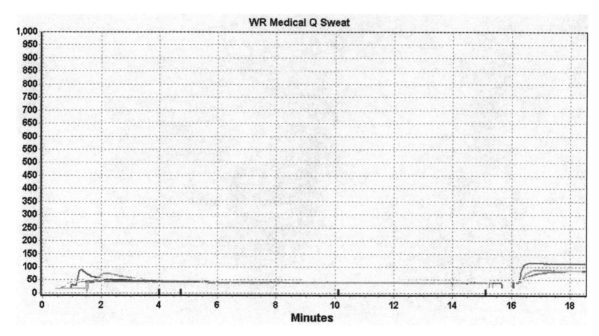

Fig. 26.3 QSART responses were absent for all sites.

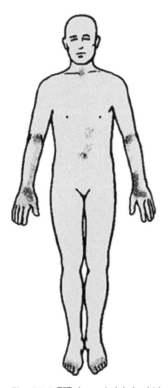

Fig. 26.4 TST showed global anhidrosis.

27 Hypothalamic dysfunction

History

A 40-year-old male with a history of craniopharyngioma treated by surgical resection and radiotherapy developed panhypopituitarism and mild encephalopathy. He remained stable for years with multiple medications to correct his hormonal deficiencies, but then developed episodes of severe hypothermia (documented body temperatures down to 33 °C), during which he complains of being cold, does not shiver, and becomes lethargic. He has had low blood pressure since the original treatments, which has not changed.

Examination

The examination is essentially normal between episodes.

Pertinent tests

No alterations in his hormonal levels, electrolytes balance, and hematologic parameters were detected.

MRI brain: stable postoperative changes over the years, with moderate, stable radiation-induced signal changes.

TST showed global anhidrosis, with rapid rise in core temperature (Fig. 27.1).

Autonomic reflex screen: showed the presence of anhidrosis and low blood pressure, with only mild cardiosympathetic dysfunction (Figs 27.2–27.5).

Diagnosis

Loss of thermoregulation due to hypothalamic damage.

Comment

Patients like this can present in various ways. In acute events (such as trauma), the presentation is with dramatic autonomic storms. In chronic cases, such as this one, due to long-standing conditions, there is no good treatment, except supportive management. Another condition in which this presentation may be seen is advanced multiple sclerosis.

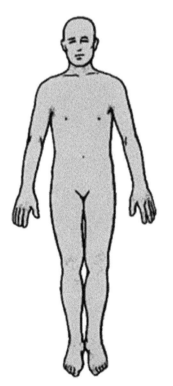

Fig. 27.1 TST showed global anhidrosis.

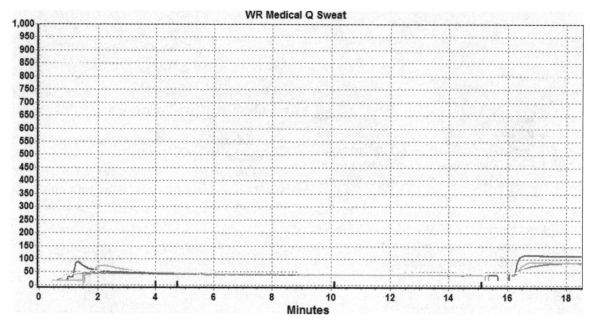

Fig. 27.2 QSART showed absent responses for all sites.

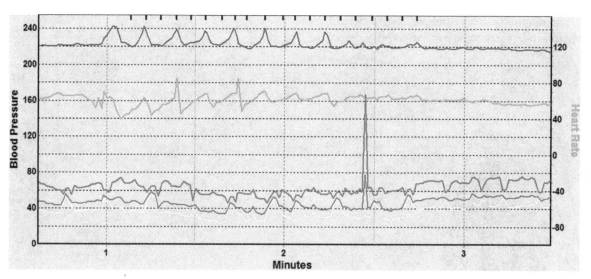

Fig. 27.3 Heart rate responses to deep breathing were normal.

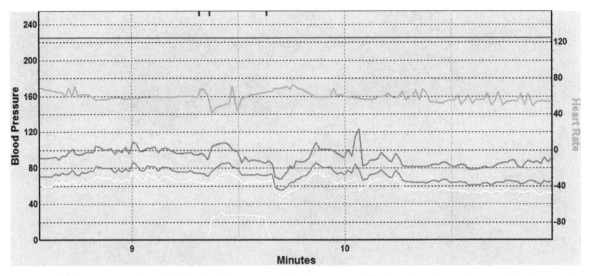

Fig. 27.4 Valsalva maneuver showed reduced cardiac responses. Blood pressure profile showed a prolonged recovery time, but no other clear-cut abnormalities.

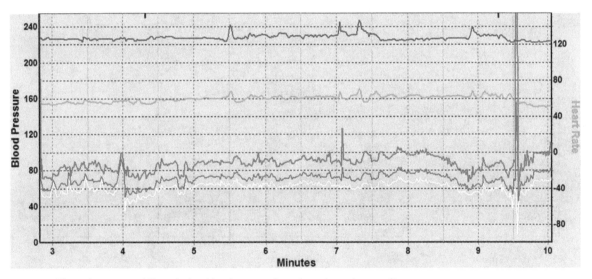

Fig. 27.5 Tilt study was normal. Note the low blood pressure throughout the entire recordings.

CASE 28 Pheochromocytoma

History

A 55-year-old male, previously healthy and fit, underwent elective surgery for hip replacement. The day after hospital dismissal, he began to experience episodes of light-headedness. Three days later he experienced syncope and was brought to a local Emergency Room. There he went into cardiac arrest due to torsades de pointes. He was successfully

89

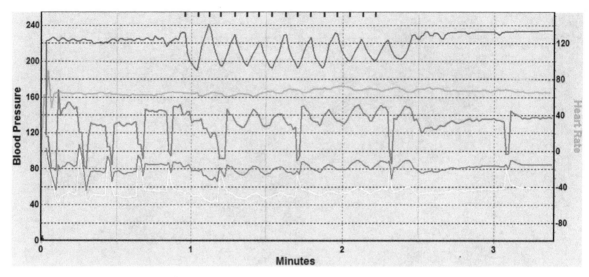

Fig. 28.1 Heart rate response to deep breathing was reduced.

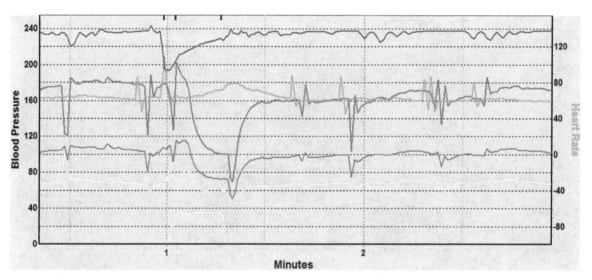

Fig. 28.2 Valsalva maneuver: cardiac responses are attenuated while blood pressure profile shows absence of late phase II and IV and slight prolongation of recovery time.

resuscitated and noted to be hypertensive (BP 244/182 mmHg). He was transferred to a tertiary center and his evaluations concluded he had long QT. Throughout his evaluations, he continued to experience extreme labile blood pressure, with both very high and very low readings. Because of continuing episodes of ventricular tachycardia despite medications, an implantable cardioverter defibrillator (ICD) was placed. He was prescribed a beta-blocker and he was then transferred to our institutions for further evaluation.

Upon admission, he was found to be anemic (Hb 9.8 g/dL), ER was elevated at 82, his other laboratory tests (electrolytes, routine chemistry group, thyroid function, protein immunofixation, autoimmune panel, and urine test) were unremarkable. ECG showed a long QT/QTc (516/520 ms). Echocardiogram showed only grade 1 of 4 left ventricular diastolic dysfunction consistent with low normal filling pressure.

Examination

His neurologic exam was normal.

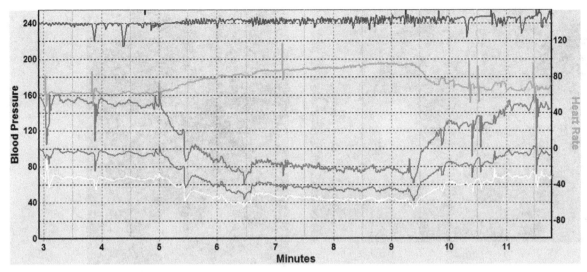

Fig. 28.3 Tilt study showed severe orthostatic hypotension with inadequate compensatory tachycardia.

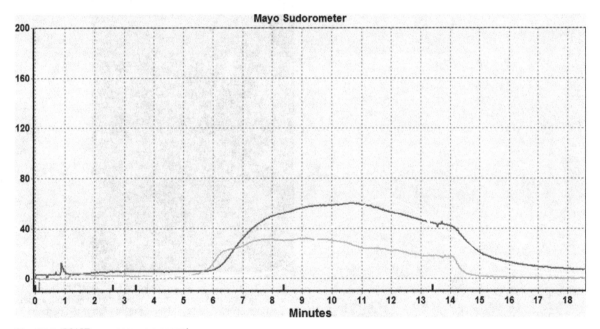

Fig. 28.4 QSART responses were normal.

Pertinent tests

Because of the history suggestive of orthostatic hypotension (OH), an autonomic reflex screen was obtained which showed severe OH and medication- and pacemaker-related blunted cardiac responses (Figs 28.1–28.4).

TST was normal.

A 24-hour urine collection showed total metanephrine level > 14 000 µg/24 h (normal < 1300 hypertensive subject), > 1000 norepinephrine (normal < 80), VMA was 57 mg/24 h (normal < 8). CT showed a large retroperitoneal mass (Fig. 28.5) that on subsequent [I^{131}]-meta-iodobenzylguanidine [MIBG] scan showed intense uptake (Fig. 28.6). The diagnosis of pheochromocytoma was made. The patient was first stabilized with alpha-blockers, volume expansion, and iron supplements before undergoing successful resection. His hormonal levels, hemodynamic parameters,

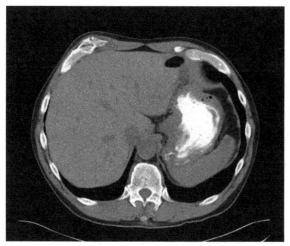

Fig. 28.5 CT abdomen showed the presence of a large retroperitoneal mass.

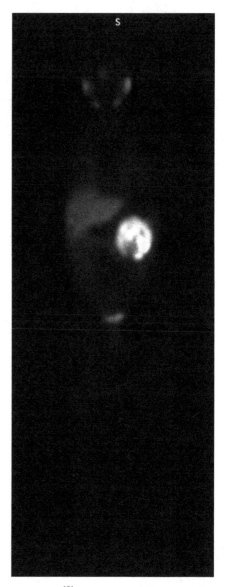

Fig. 28.6 [I¹³¹]-MIBG scan. Whole body 24 h planar imaging. SPECT/CT imaging of the abdomen. The huge left abdominal mass shows intense MIBG uptake in the lobulated soft tissue portions surrounding an inactive central pseudocyst.

and ECG normalized and the ICD/pacemaker was removed 1 month after surgery. He required no further treatment.

Comment

Pheochromocytoma can cause long QT and a variety of arrhythmias due to the sympathetic surge. Orthostatic hypotension is quite typical as well, owing to volume depletion. That, combined with the release of catecholamines, can account for the extremely labile blood pressure. The anemia was likely due to a combination of blood loss at surgery, hemorrhage into the tumor mass (seen on CT), and iron deficiency from the patient's vegetarian diet.

Syncope

History

A 19-year-old female presented for evaluation of recurrent syncope, fatigue, and pain. She reported having a long-standing problem with orthostatic light-headedness. Episodes of stress or fatigue would trigger or worsen these episodes. She was diagnosed also with vasovagal episodes and her parents reported numerous occasions when this type of syncope occurred. Pain and stress could easily trigger an attack. At the age of 16 years she had a prolonged event with convulsive activity. Brain MRI and EEG were normal. The year prior to presentation she had a particularly stressful experience while abroad and her symptoms appeared to intensify, with increase in severity and frequency. She also began to complain of difficulty concentrating and became unable to exercise owing to light-headedness, shortness of breath, fatigue, and diffuse pain. She underwent extensive cardiologic evaluations, including echocardiogram and Holter monitoring that were unremarkable, but on a tilt study an episode of neurocardiogenic syncope was recorded.

She had no other autonomic symptom except for constipation. Her review of system was significant for episodes suspicious for cataplexy – a condition her father also suffers from.

Examination

The examination was normal, but she suffered a spell while sitting in the physician's office, characterized by loss of consciousness followed by myoclonic jerking, not resolved by laying the patient supine, but spontaneously stopping after approximately 30 seconds.

Pertinent tests

Her autonomic testing was normal (Figs 29.1–29.2 and 29.4), but during tilt she experienced one of her spells and the ECG showed a 20-second asystole (Fig. 29.3a, b). She underwent pacemaker placement with excellent results.

Comment

Syncope is common and unless recurrent, is usually not disabling or malignant. Unless captured on recording, it may be impossible to differentiate the type on history alone. The evaluation and management of syncope can be extremely tedious and frustrating as it may take a long time to capture the right spell, as in this case. Furthermore, some arrhythmias can be caused by seizure activity and only simultaneous recording may discriminate between ictal (i.e.

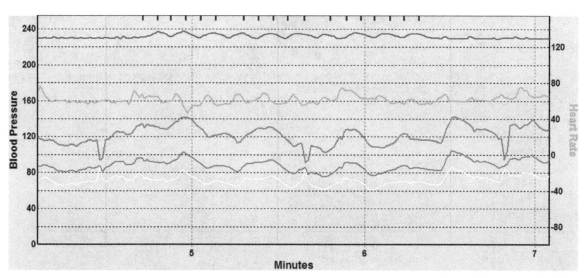

Fig. 29.1 Heart rate response to deep breathing was normal.

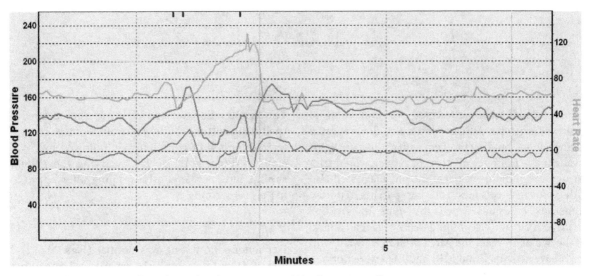

Fig. 29.2 Valsalva maneuver showed normal cardiac responses and blood pressure profile.

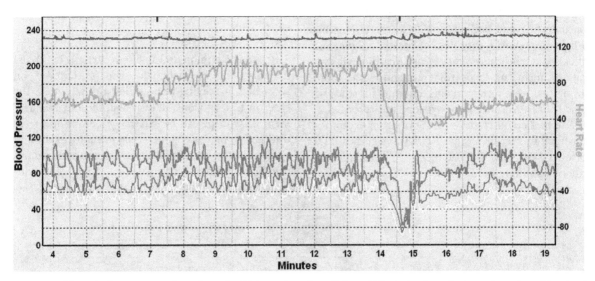

Fig. 29.3a Tilt study: there was excessive tachycardia with hemodynamic oscillations. At 7 minutes the patient experienced a sudden drop in heart rate followed by a drop in blood pressure and syncope occurred.

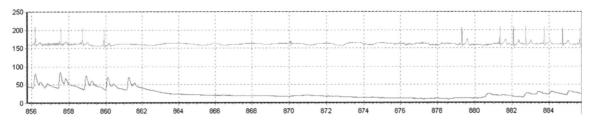

Fig. 29.3b ECG strip of the event demonstrated the 20 second asystole.

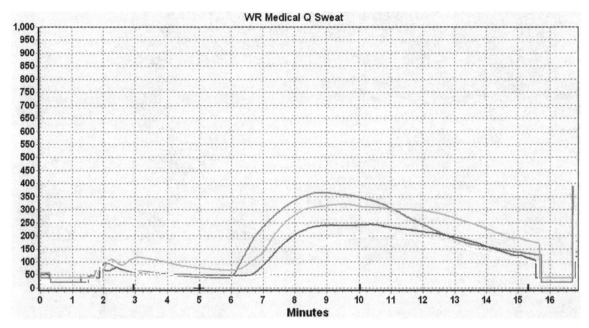

WR Medical Q Sweat

Minutes

Fig. 29.4 QSART responses were normal for all sites.

epileptic) syncope and convulsive syncope due to hypoperfusion caused by the arrhythmia.

While some brief pauses (2–3 seconds) can be seen in other forms of syncope and do not require any invasive intervention, in this case the length of asystole prompted an aggressive management to prevent not only more simple syncope episodes (that the patient also had) but mainly to avoid ischemic brain injury.

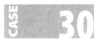

30 Harlequin's syndrome

History

A 44-year-old female presented with a history of flushing affecting the left forehead. This was relatively mild at first. Over the next 5 years, the episodes recurred consistently but became more severe and were associated with significant unilateral sweating. The episodes were precipitated by exercise and by raised ambient heat. Occasionally, there might be an emotional component, but this is rather questionable. The sweating would begin in her forehead, extend to her cheek and chin. She noticed beads of sweating in the same distribution. Over time, this has extended to the left upper chest in the infraclavicular area. She had no other autonomic symptoms. She had a history of migraine; however, this affected chiefly the right side and with no autonomic manifestations.

Examination

The examination, while asymptomatic, was normal.

95

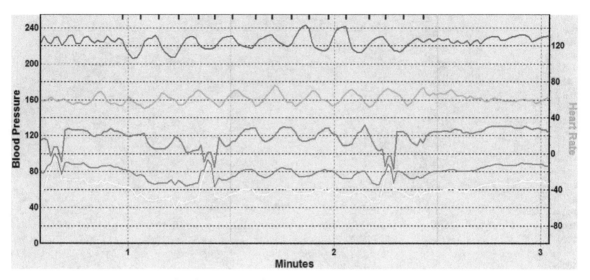

Fig. 30.1 Heart rate response to deep breathing was normal.

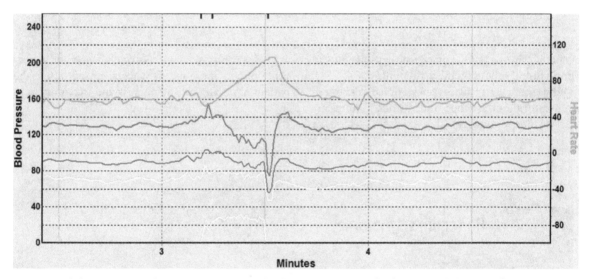

Fig. 30.2 Valsalva maneuver: cardiac responses are normal, but the blood pressure profile showed a slight blunting of late phase II.

Pertinent tests

Hematologic, endocrine, routine chemistry, and neuroimmunology panel were normal.

MRI of the brain, cervical and thoracic spine was normal.

The autonomic screen showed evidence of vasomotor insufficiency (blunted late phase II BP response during Valsalva and initial drop on tilt-up) (Figs 30.1–30.3), and there was a tendency to excessive orthostatic tachycardia. There was an absent sweat response over the right forearm, but normal on the left (Fig. 30.4 a, b).

In addition two more responses were measured in the subclavicular areas and the response on the left was much larger and had persistent sweat activity, indicating an overactive system (Fig. 30.5: green line left, red right).

TST: there was asymmetric sweat over the face (Figs 30.6–30.7), with reduction on the right and excessive sweat on the left. There was also right foot

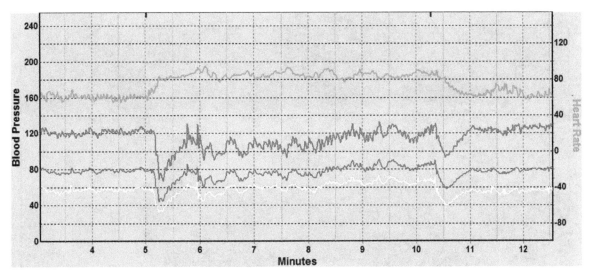

Fig. 30.3 Tilt study showed initial orthostatic hypotension with rapid recovery.

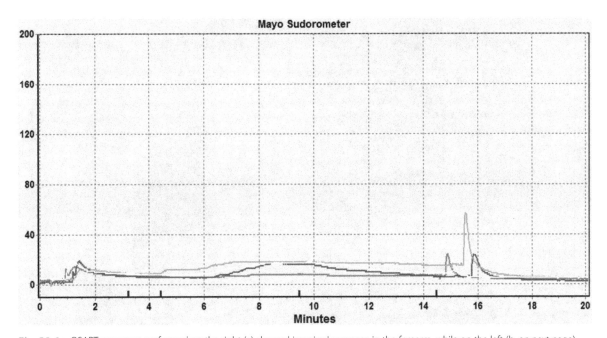

Fig. 30.4a QSART responses performed on the right (a) showed impaired response in the forearm, while on the left (b, on next page) responses were normal for all sites.

and leg sweat reduction. Flushing of the left side of the face only was noted after she showered (Fig. 30.8).

She was therefore diagnosed with Harlequin's syndrome – an idiopathic sympathetic lesion proximal to the carotid bifurcation with contralateral compensatory hyperhidrosis.

She underwent a stellate ganglion block to control the flushing, which was successful. Since then,

however, she continued to progress with more generalized anhidrosis, and she began to experience mild orthostatic intolerance.

Repeat testing identified low-titer positivity for the AchR autoantibody. TST showed progression of the abnormalities noted before (Fig. 30.9).

She was treated symptomatically for the orthostatic symptoms with pyridostigmine and

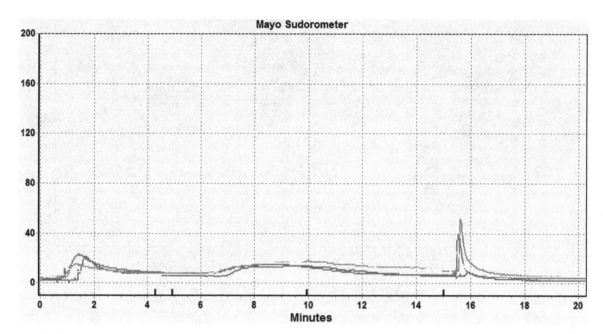

Fig. 30.4b (cont.)

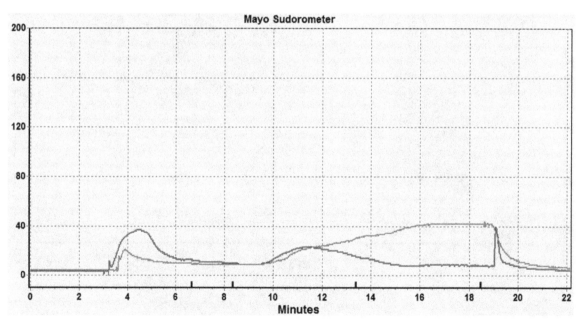

Fig. 30.5 QSART measured over the supraclavicular regions showed larger sweat response with persistent sweat activity over the left (green tracing) compared with the right (red tracing).

returned 2 years later with essentially unchanged symptoms.

Repeat testing showed again low-titer positivity for the AchR autoantibody (0.13 nmol/mL, normal < 0.02), with slight improvement in her autonomic testing and sweat test (Fig. 30.10).

Comment

Harlequin's syndrome is idiopathic in most cases. It is unclear in this case if this was the first manifestation of a more generalized, albeit patchy, limited auto-immune form (see also Case 31).

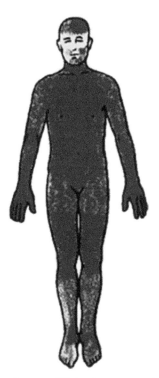

Fig. 30.6 TST showing asymmetric sweat over the face, with reduced production on the right and excessive on the left.

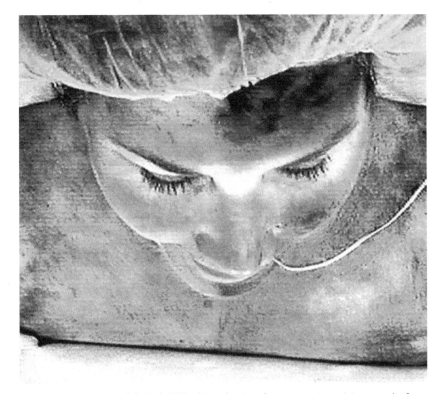

Fig. 30.7 Image taken while in the TST cabinet showing the asymmetric sweating over the face.

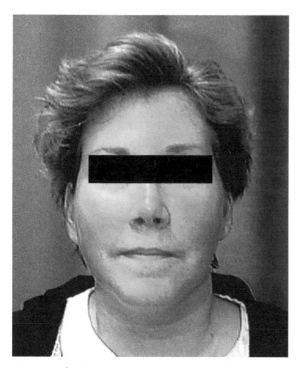

Fig. 30.8 After the patient showered, asymmetric flushing was noted.

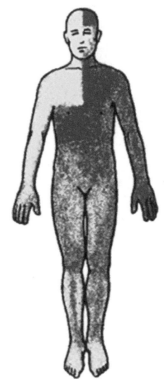

Fig. 30.9 TST showed the progression of the autonomic neuro-pathy with now widespread, albeit patchy anhidrosis superimposed on the regional anhidrosis over the right side.

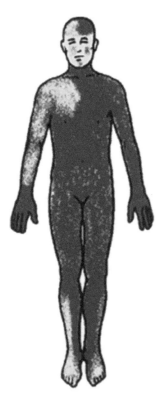

Fig. 30.10 TST showing mild improvement in the patient's auto-immune neuropathy.

History

A 64-year-old female presented 5 months after the acute onset of blurry vision with midriasis. The patient reported headache at the onset that had also persisted since. She complained of mild light-headedness with prolonged standing and noticed mild gait imbalance. She reported she did not sweat anymore since the onset of the visual symptoms. She had pre-existent irritable bowel syndrome and occasional stress incontinence that had not changed. There was no xerostomia or xerophthalmia.

Examination

She had Adie's pupils. She had absent ankle reflexes and sensory loss, worse to large fiber modalities, up to her ankles. She had a positive Romberg maneuver and difficulty with tandem gait.

Pertinent tests

Her routine laboratory tests showed a borderline low vitamin B12 level (with normal methylmalonic acid level), but were otherwise normal, including a negative hematologic, endocrine, connective tissue disorder, and neuroimmunology panel. She had extensive testing, including MRI of brain and spine, that also were normal.

Autonomic testing was impacted by the patient having a cough, but showed only mild impairment of cardiac responses while vasomotor and postganglionic sudomotor functions were intact (Figs 31.1–31.4).

TST showed global anhidrosis, suggesting a preganglionic or ganglionic process (Fig. 31.5).

The patient was diagnosed with idiopathic cholinergic failure consistent with the clinical diagnosis of Ross' syndrome.

Comment

Ross' syndrome is classically described as the triad of segmental anhidrosis, tonic pupils, and areflexia. But as for Case 30, the phenotype and clinical course can be variable. This case has global anhidrosis, and may suggest these "idiopathic" forms are in fact limited autoimmune autonomic ganglionopathies. Harlequin's syndrome may be one as well.

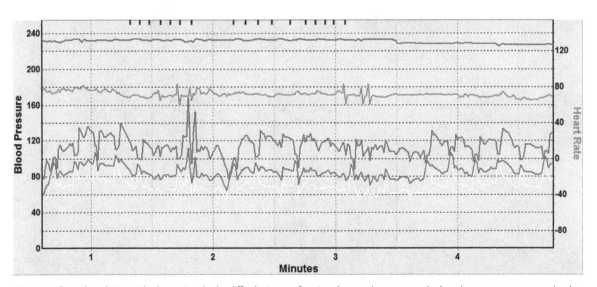

Fig. 31.1 Deep breathing study: the patient had a difficult time performing the test due to a cough, thus the responses appeared to be almost absent. They were nonetheless attenuated.

101

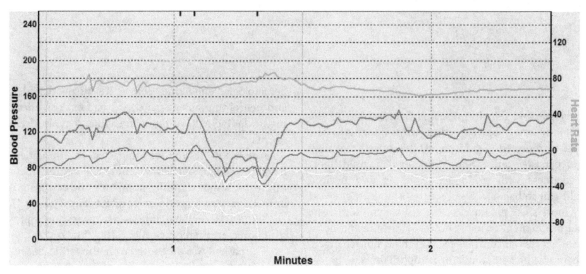

Fig. 31.2 Valsalva maneuver showed reduction of cardiac responses. Blood pressure profile showed an attenuated phase IV but was otherwise normal for age.

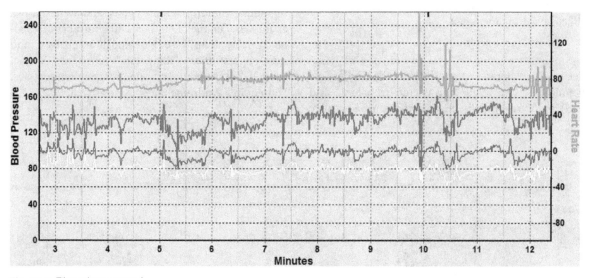

Fig. 31.3 Tilt study was normal.

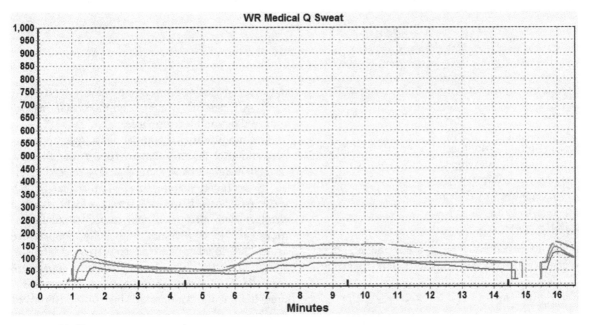

Fig. 31.4 QSART responses were normal.

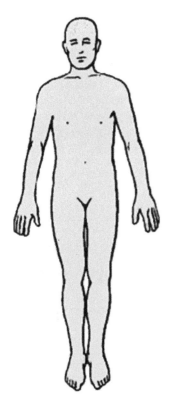

Fig. 31.5 TST showed global anhidrosis.

Autoimmune encephalopathy with autonomic manifestations

History

A 27-year-old male presented with a 2–3 year history of irritability, night sweats, 52 kg weight loss and 1 year of episodic vomiting with severe constipation. He subsequently developed neurologic symptoms characterized by fluctuating incoordination, oscillopsia, and cognitive impairment.

Examination

The exam revealed an amnestic syndrome, multifocal myoclonus, diffuse hyperreflexia, ataxia, and nystagmus.

Pertinent tests

Gastrointestinal motility studies documented gastroparesis and bowel hypomotility.

Autonomic reflex testing demonstrated cardiovagal and vasomotor dysfunction (Figs 32.1–32.4).

Video EEG demonstrated continuous tremulousness (which was confirmed by surface EMG to be myoclonus) without epileptiform correlate.

His neuroimmunology panel detected a serum-specific IgG for dipeptidyl-peptidase-like protein-6 (DPP6, a.k.a. DPPX).

The symptoms improved after treatment with intravenous methylprednisolone. Oral prednisone

and a steroid-sparing immunosuppressant (mycophenolate) were added. Weight, cognition, and balance improved but did not normalize.

Five months after the initial neurologic presentation, and after discontinuing corticosteroid therapy, visual hallucinations developed, and were accompanied by profound diaphoresis, hypothermia (34 °C), and leukocytosis. No infection was evident. Cardiac arrest ensued; after successful resuscitation, fluctuations of blood pressure and body temperature (from 29 °C to 40 °C) necessitated extended intensive care. Diaphoresis, blood pressure, and temperature normalized following intravenous methylprednisolone treatment. Autonomic instability improved greatly after plasma exchange, rituximab, and slowly tapered prednisone therapy, but ataxia, disrupted sleep, and excessive daytime somnolence continued, with residual cognitive impairment, and urinary retention due to an atonic bladder.

Comment

DPPX is a regulatory subunit of the voltage-gated A-type (rapidly inactivating) Kv4.2 potassium channel complex expressed in neuronal dendrites and soma. Kv4.2 is the principal channel responsible for transient, inhibitory currents in the central and

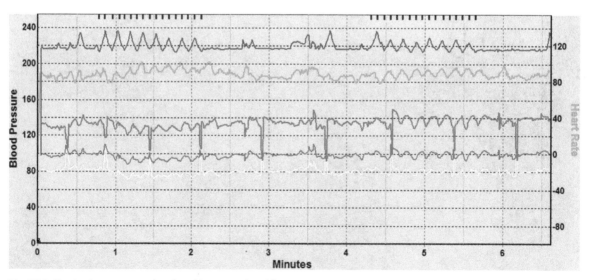

Fig. 32.1 Heart rate response to deep breathing was reduced for age.

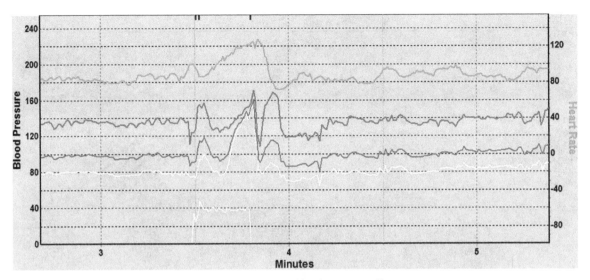

Fig. 32.2 Valsalva maneuver showed normal cardiac responses and blood pressure profile.

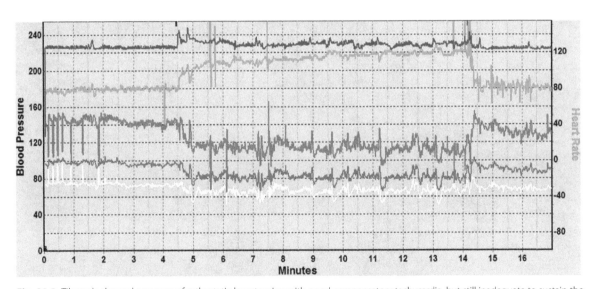

Fig. 32.3 Tilt study showed presence of orthostatic hypotension with good compensatory tachycardia, but still inadequate to sustain the blood pressure.

peripheral nervous systems. Recent reports identified few patients positive for such antibody that presented with a multifocal, hyper-excitable encephalitic phenotype. The disorder is less common than the autoimmune NMDA receptor encephalitis. Experience is still limited, but the condition is often severe, tends to relapse but responds to immunotherapy, which should be promptly started.

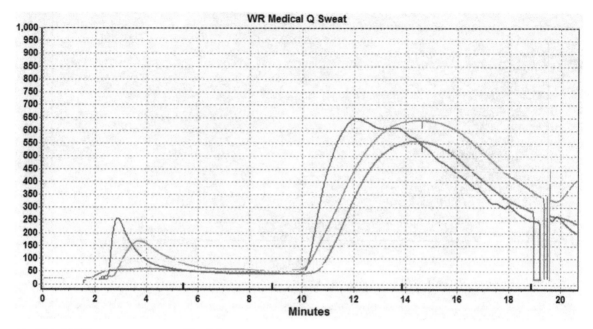

Fig. 32.4 QSART responses were normal for all sites.

Vignettes

Vignette 1

Tilt-up study of a dehydrated patient (due to diarrhea). Upon tilt-up, there is pulse pressure compression and gradual decline in blood pressure with a compensatory, robust heart rate response. Such pattern should not be confused with inappropriate tachycardia, where there is no decrement in blood pressure although there may be pulse pressure compression.

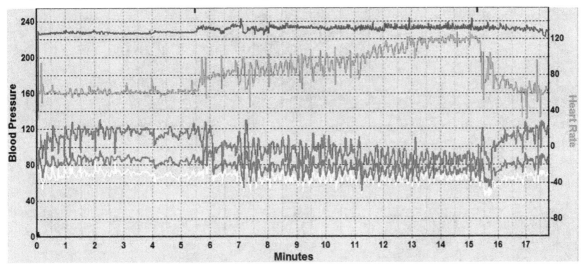

Vignette 2

Valsalva maneuver of the same patient as the above tilt. Again, notice the pulse pressure compression and mild reduction in late phase II of the maneuver indicating mild vasoconstriction insufficiency.

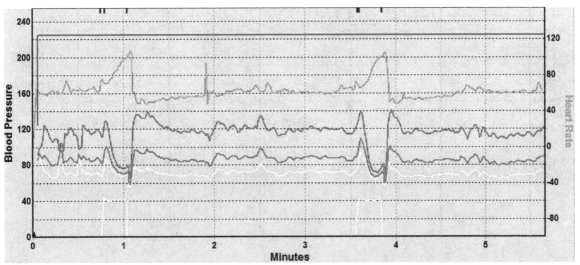

Vignette 3

Tilt-up study in three subjects with mild orthostatic intolerance. There are prominent hemodynamic oscillations accompanied, or likely induced, by hyperventilation (notice blue line profile). Hyperventilation: the oscillations in heart rate and blood pressure, mimicking OI/POTS pattern, are induced by hyperventilation in these anxious patients.

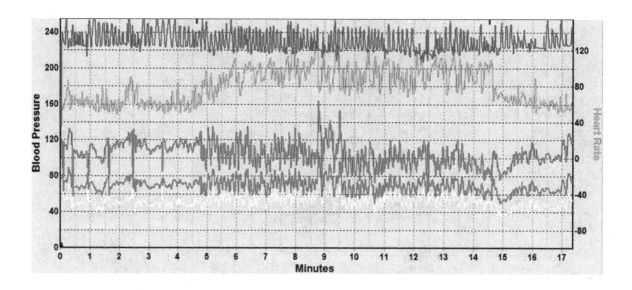

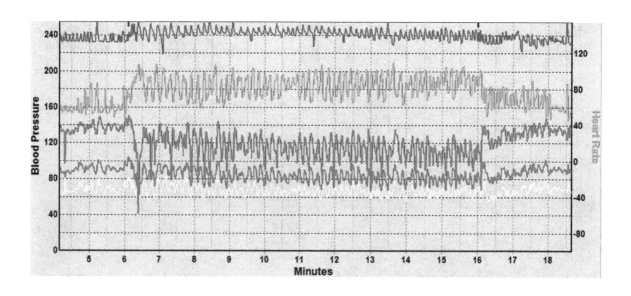

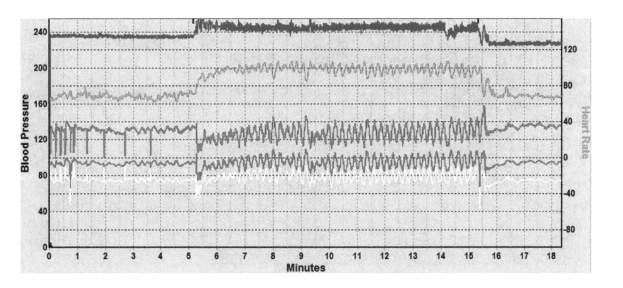

Vignette 4

Tilt-up study in subjects with severe pain (a, b). Standing exacerbated the pain causing the excessive tachycardic response. Another example (c) of the effect of pain and talking when tilted up.

(a)

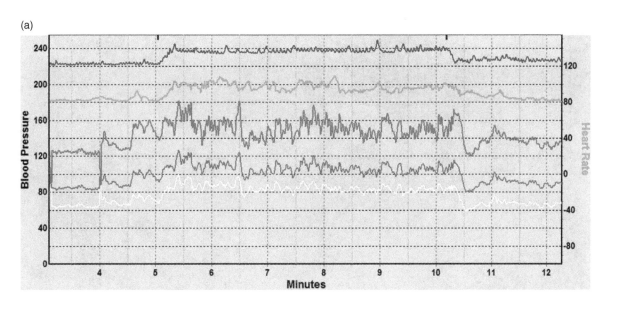

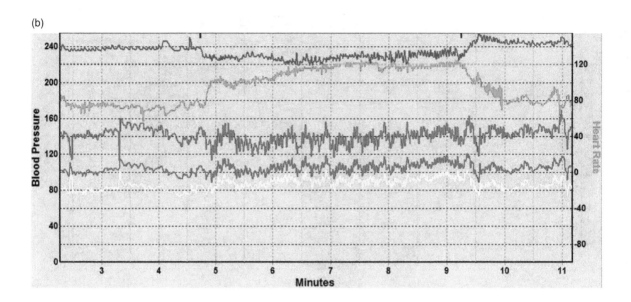

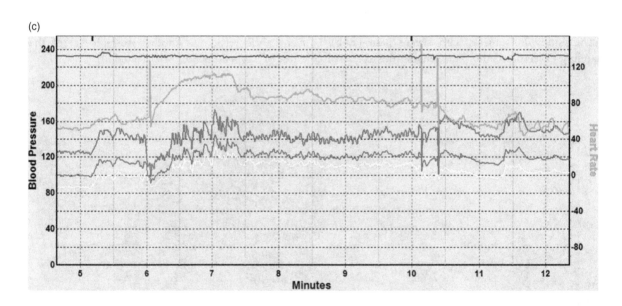

Vignettes

Vignette 5

An example of an autonomic neuropathy affecting cardiovagal and cardiosympathetic functions while vasomotor function was still intact. The opposite may occur as well.

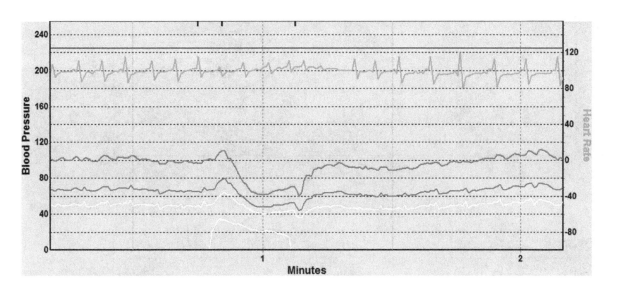

Vignette 6

Effect of CO_2 washout during deep breathing (a): heart rate increases and variability is reduced. (b, c) Another example in which the responses normalize after the patient relaxed. This was due to a combination of sympathetic activation and CO_2 washout. (d) Another example.

(a)

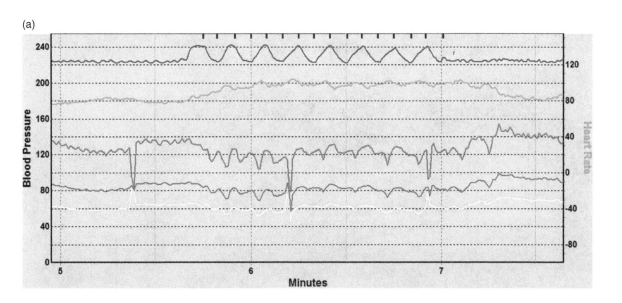

(b)

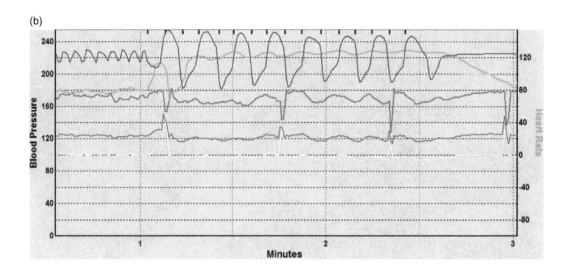

(c)

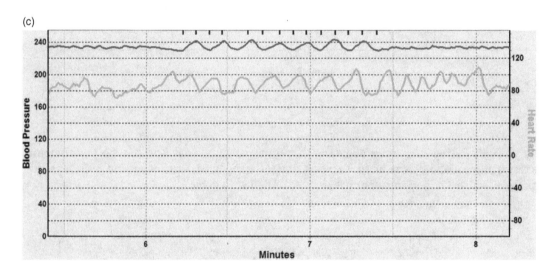

(d)

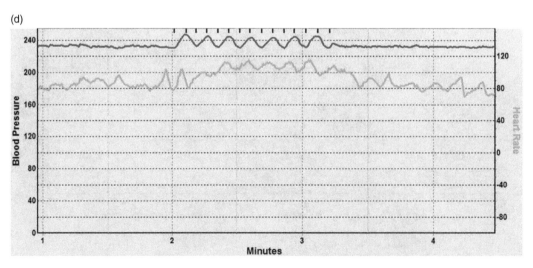

Vignette 7

During the study, a patient with a history of spells experienced one of his spells characterized by flushing and feeling unwell: his heart rate and blood pressure at that time spiked. The whole episode lasted less than 1 minute. The patient did not lose consciousness, and was fully lucid during the episode. The nature of these spells remains unclear, but they manifest as a "mini" autonomic storm.

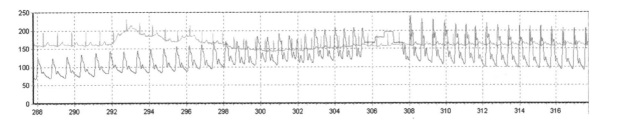

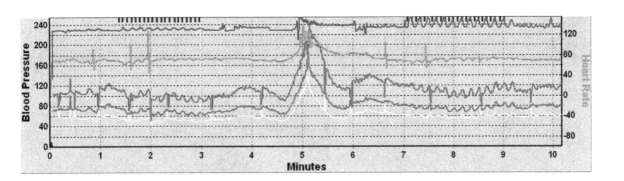

Vignette 8

AAG series (8.1a–d): severe AAG: here we have profound impairment of cardioacceleration but less severe vasoconstrictor failure. QSART shows preserved sweating in the forearm, markedly reduced but still present sweat in the proximal leg and absent responses at the distal sites. The pattern is one of global cardiovagal, baroreflex, and sympathetic (cardiac, vasomotor, and postganglionic sudomotor) failure. Another case (8.2a–f), before (8.2a–c) and after (8.2d–f) IVIG treatment: on deep breathing cardiac responses are markedly diminished indicating cardiovagal impairment. Both Valsalva and tilt show profound vasomotor failure, with absence of late phase BP recovery, slow recovery to baseline BP and absent phase IV overshoot. Cardioacceleration was still valid. On tilt, dramatic orthostatic hypotension prompts quick tilt back. After 6 weeks of treatment, although the study is still abnormal, significant improvement can be appreciated in heart rate response during deep breathing and vasomotor function is recovering as well, allowing the patient to tolerate the standing posture for 10 minutes. Another example before (8.3a–c) and after (8.3d–f) treatment: this case shows the most dramatic improvement after treatment.

(8.1a)

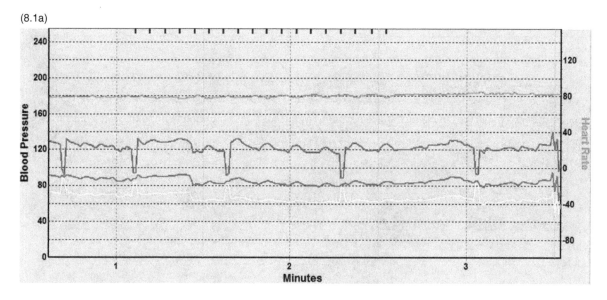

(8.1b)

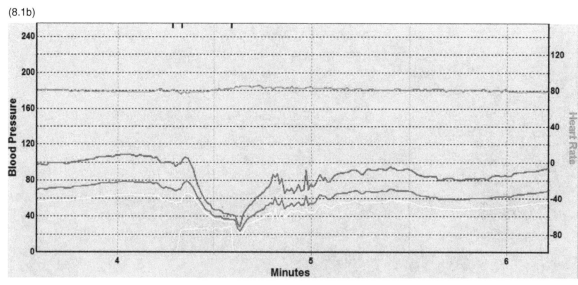

(8.1c)

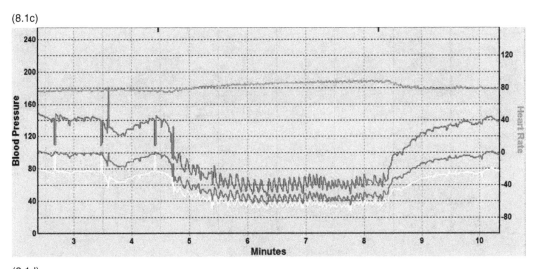

(8.1d)

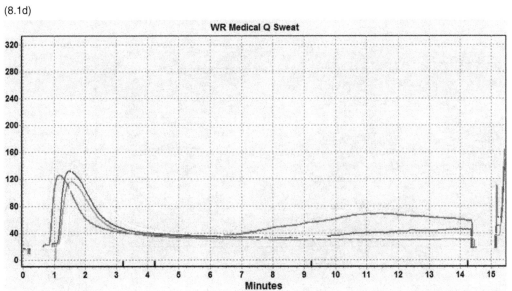

(8.2a)

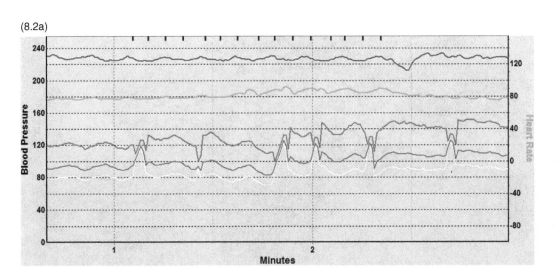

(8.2b)

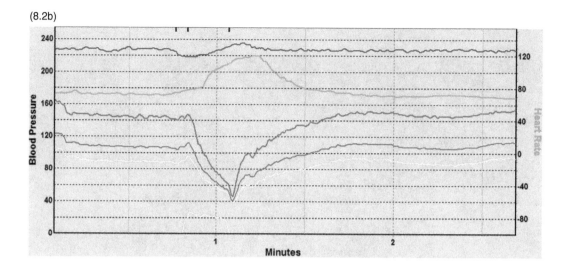

(8.2c)

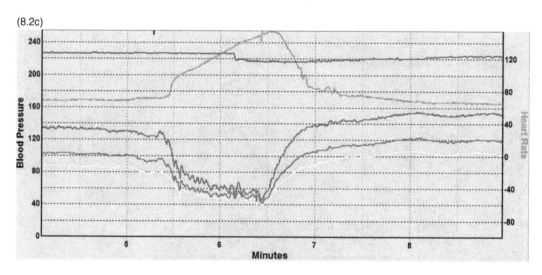

(8.2d)

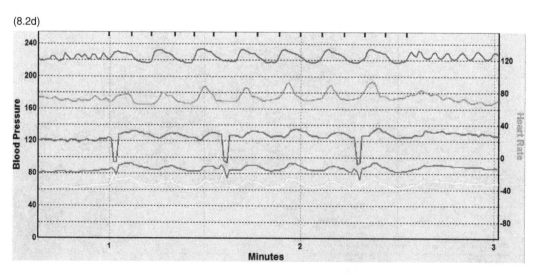

(8.2e)

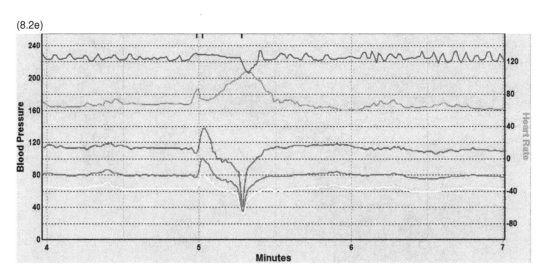

(8.2f)

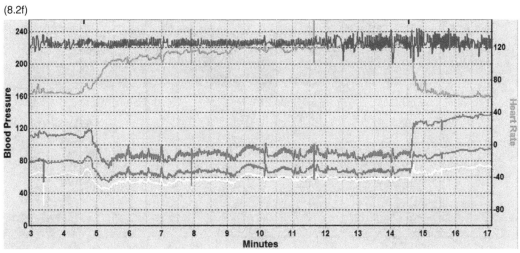

(8.3a)

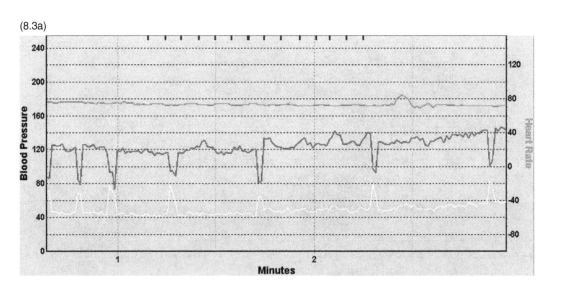

(8.3b)

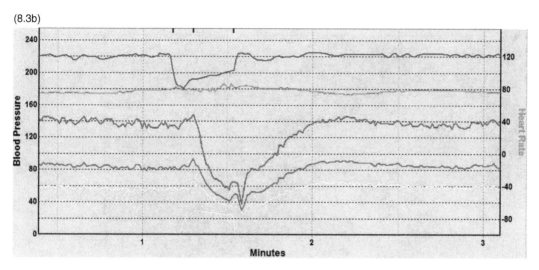

(8.3c)

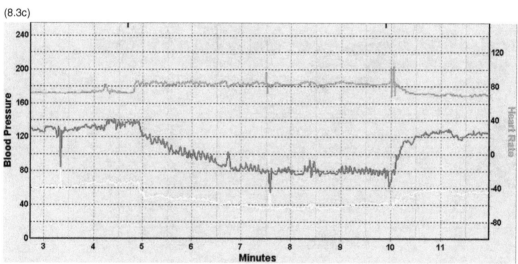

(8.3d)

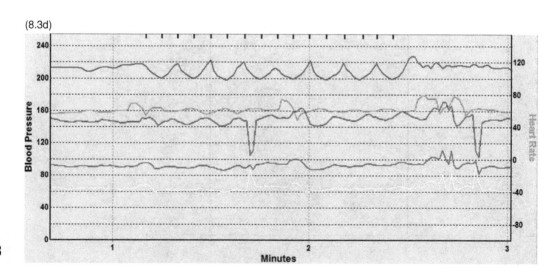

(8.3e)

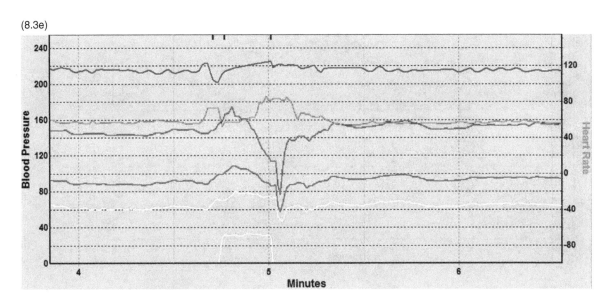

(8.3f)

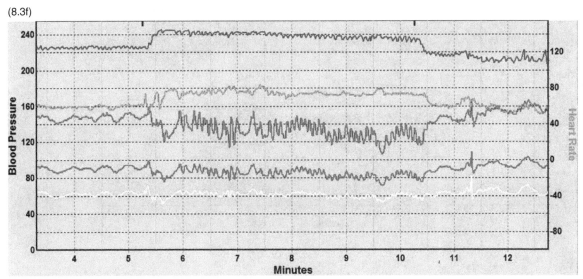

Vignette 9

Amyloidosis (9.1a–d and 9.2a–d) – the testing demonstrates the classic profile of cardiac autonomic neuropathy. Direct myocardial involvement may also account for these findings. Note the absence of HR variability during DB and VM and vasoconstrictor insufficiency on Valsalva (very small late phase II recovery, markedly prolonged BP recovery to baseline and no phase IV overshoot present) and on tilt, resulting in orthostatic hypotension. QSART is still preserved, in this specific case. Amyloidosis with CHF (9.3 and 9.4): heart rate tracing has been eliminated as it showed just atrial fibrillation. The blood pressure profile during Valsalva does not change when comparing the first maneuver (supine) with the subsequent ones done at 20, 30 and 40 degree bed tilt in an attempt to eliminate the flat-top profile. Such a pattern is observed in CHF and indicated lack of heart chambers compliance. In normal subjects with flat-top profile, inclining the bed will at the other end elicit appearance of the more "classic" Valsalva maneuver BP profile.

119

(9.1a)

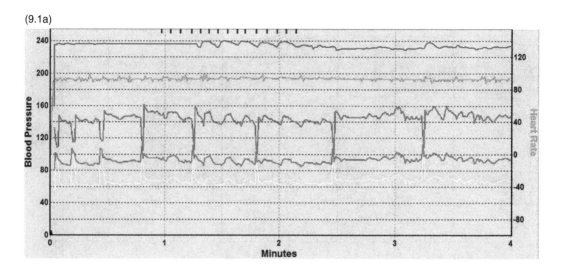

(9.1b)

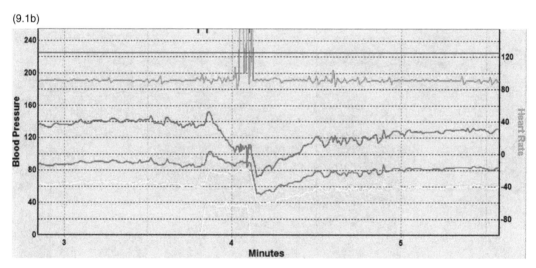

(9.1c)

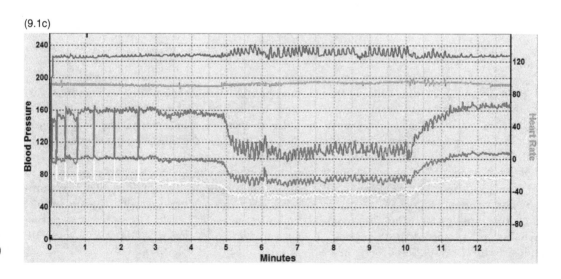

(9.1d)

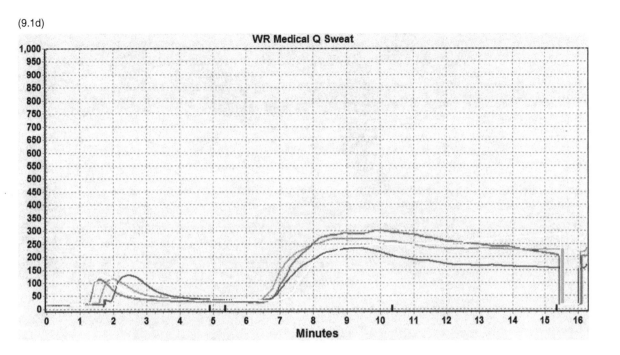

(9.2a)

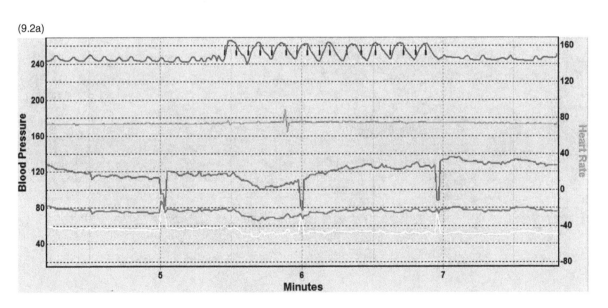

(9.2b)

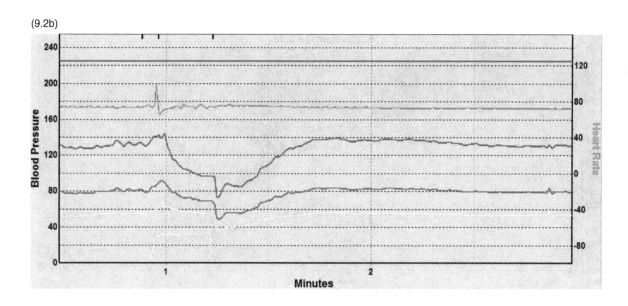

(9.2c)

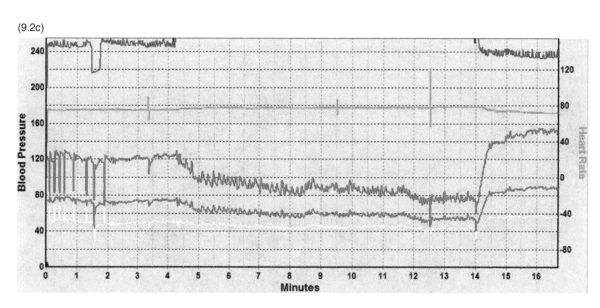

(9.2d)

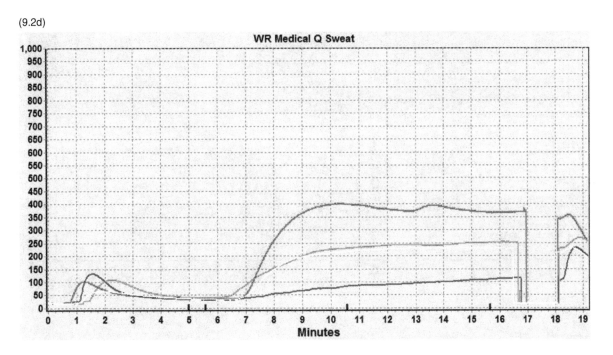

(9.3)

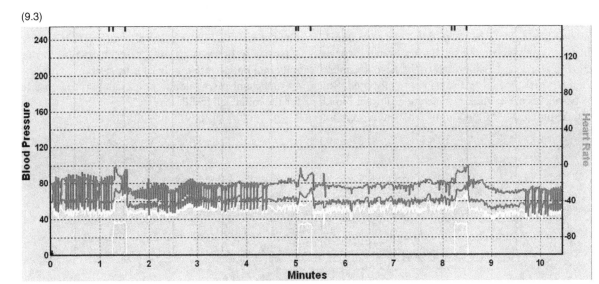

(9.4)

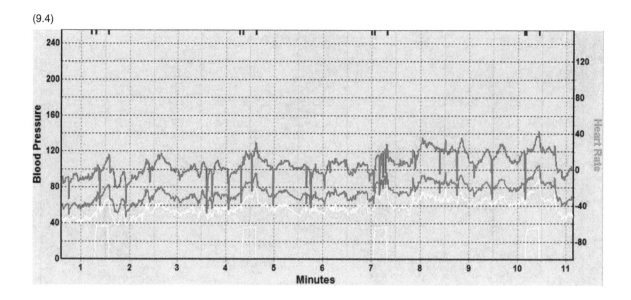

Vignette 10

Baroreflex failure due to prior RT to the neck: heart rate responses to deep breathing are preserved, baroreflexes play only a minor role in generating sinus arrhythmia, which is mainly generated by Hering-Breuer (stretch lung receptors) and Bainbridge (right heart chamber filling sensors) reflexes and vagal nerve mediated. But the baroflexes are critical to generate a normal blood pressure profile during the Valsalva maneuver: here we have no late phase II or IV and prolonged recovery time with inadequate cardiac response. During tilt, there is an initial drop in blood pressure, followed by a partial recovery suggesting vasoconstriction is not impaired but activated only later by slower compensatory mechanisms, while baroreflex failure is responsible for the initial fall in BP.

(10a)

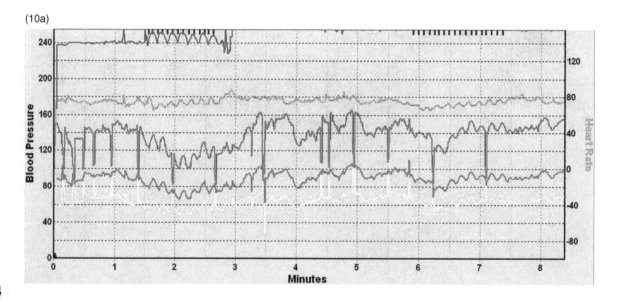

(10b)

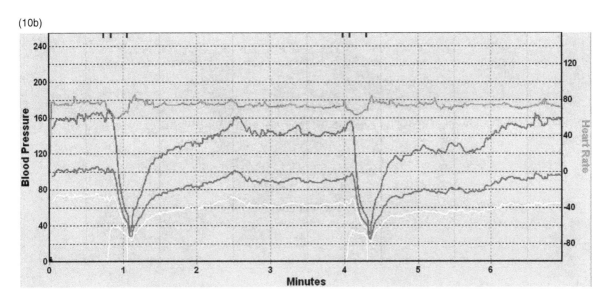

(10c)

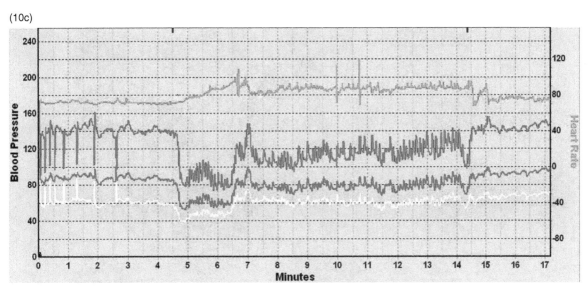

Vignette 11

POTS series: hyperadrenergic type (11.1a, b): note the large phase IV overshoot at the end of Valsalva and during tilt the increase in both blood pressure and heart rate with prominent oscillations in hemodynamic parameters. POTS neuropathic (11.2a, b; 11.3a, b, two examples): During Valsalva there is only a blunted late phase II, suggesting vasoconstrictor insufficiency, likely due to limited alpha-adrenergic denervation associated with excessive HR increase during tilt. The first example also has vasodepressor syncope at end of tilt. The third case (11.3a–c) also shows the reduced QSART distally, oftentimes seen in neuropathic POTS. (11.4a, b) shows a case with vasovagal syncope (due to sudden sympathetic withdrawal in yet another POTS patient). (11.5a, b) another example of POTS, non-specific. (11.6) a classic POTS pattern during tilt. (11.7): a POTS case with prominent resting tachycardia. (11.8a, b)): a brief episode of arrhythmia was observed in this POTS patient after she was tilted back.

(11.1a)

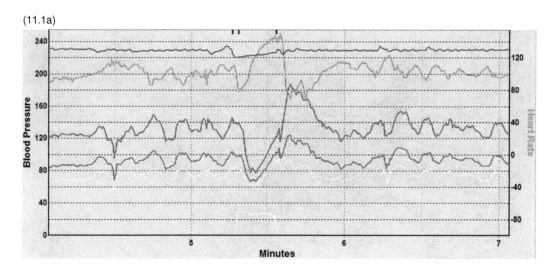

(11.1b)

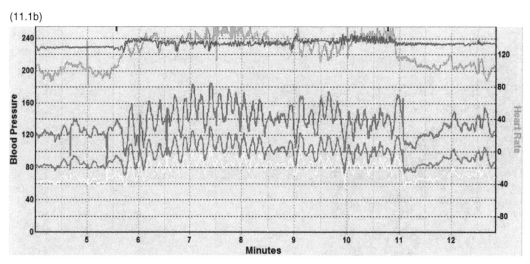

(11.2a)

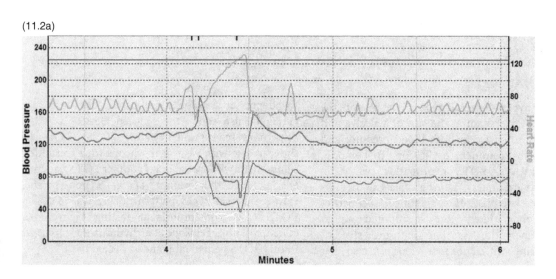

(11.2b)

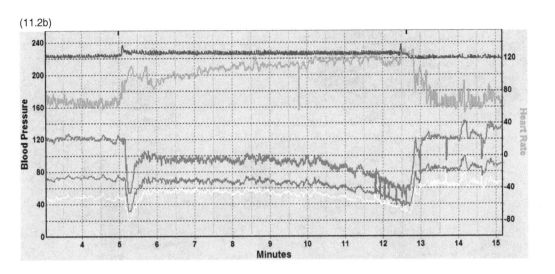

(11.3a)

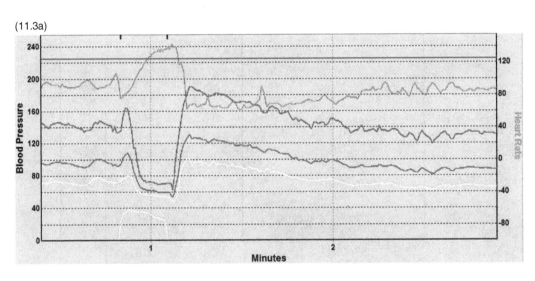

(11.3b)

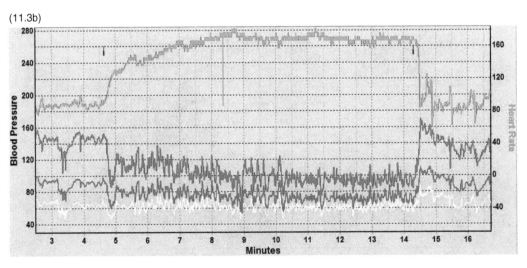

(11.3c)

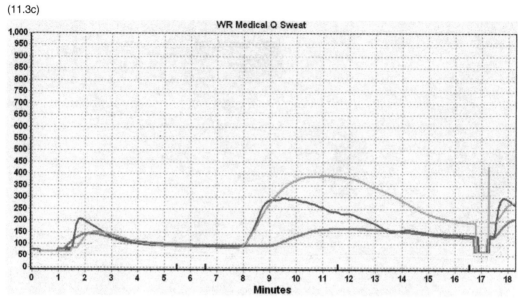

(11.4a)

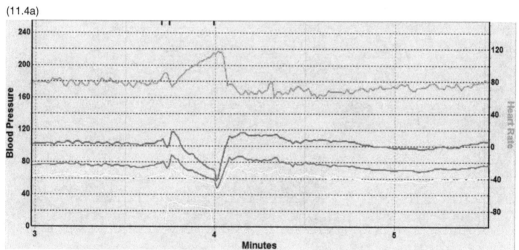

(11.4b)

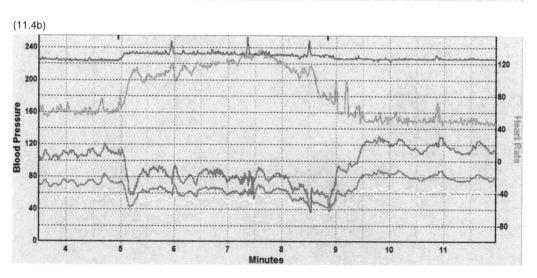

(11.5a)

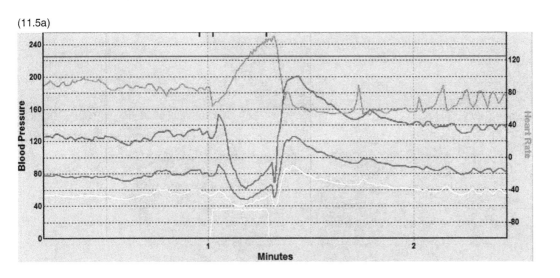

(11.5b)

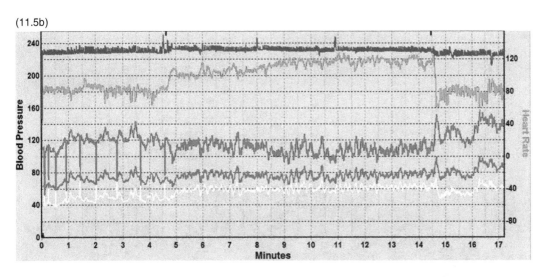

(11.6)

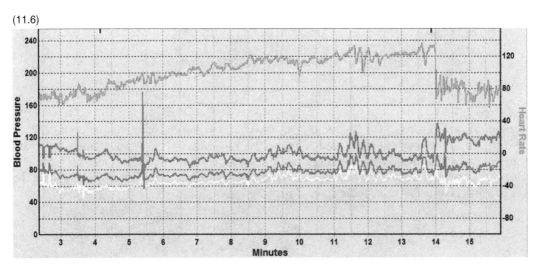

(11.7)

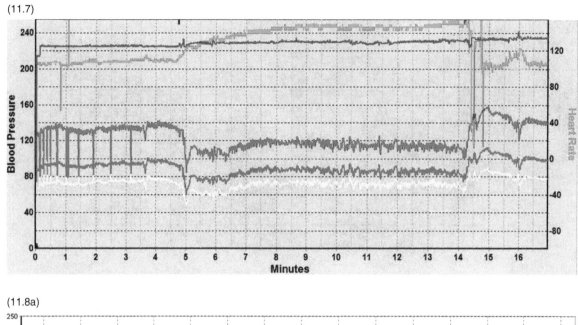

(11.8a)

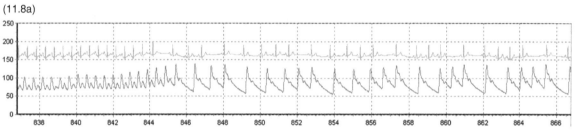

(11.8b)

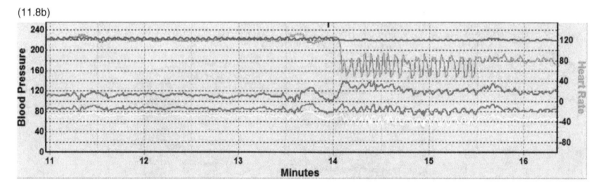

Vignette 12

Diabetic cardiac autonomic neuropathy (12.1a–d and 12.2a–c): severe loss of heart rate variability, portending poor prognosis, in patient with long-standing diabetes. During Valsalva there is loss of late phase II and IV with prolonged recovery time, indicating also vasoconstriction and baroreflex failure. On tilt, as expected, profound OH occurred. Despite the severe cardiovagal, cardiosympathetic, and sympathetic vasomotor failure, sweat responses were intact in the first case.

(12.1a)

(12.1b)

(12.1c)

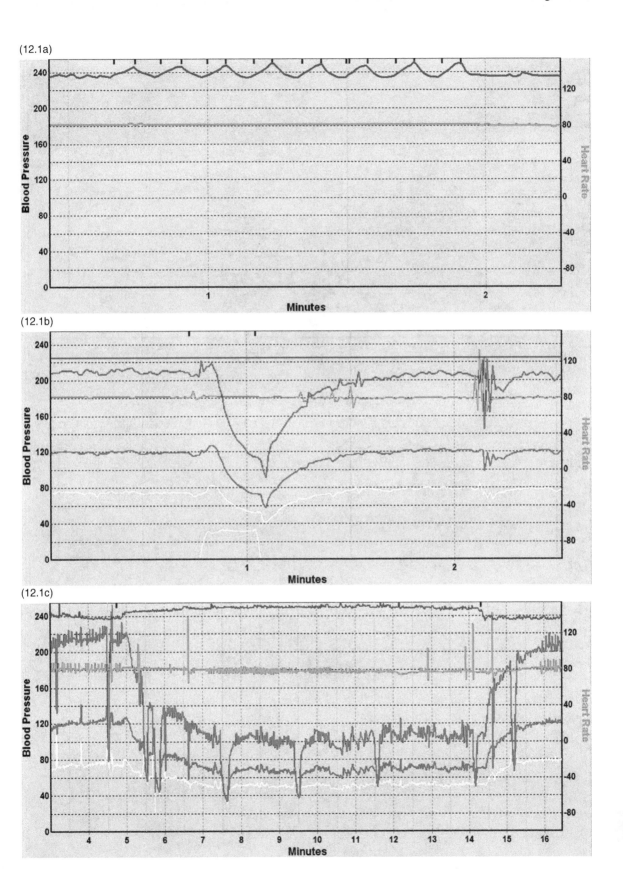

(12.1d)

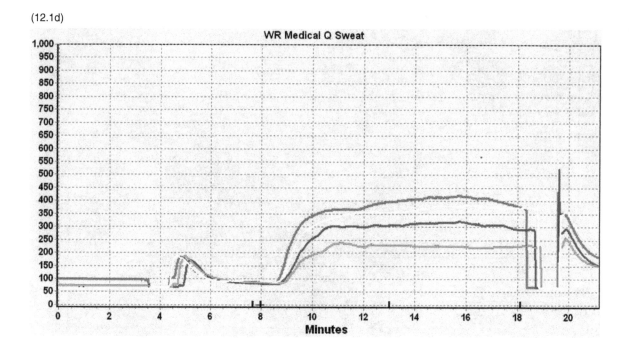

(12.2a)

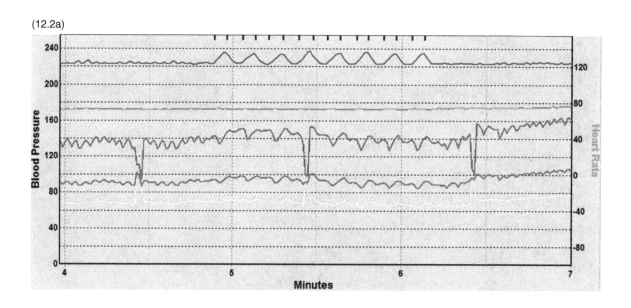

(12.2b)

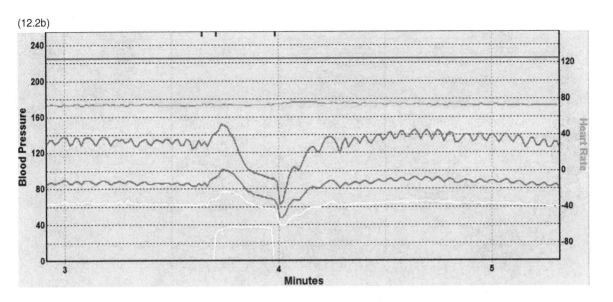

(12.2c)

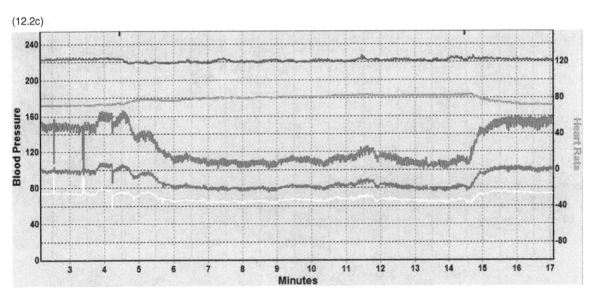

Vignette 13

A case of autonomic neuropathy of unknown etiology with severe impairment of cardiac responses and orthostatic hypotension.

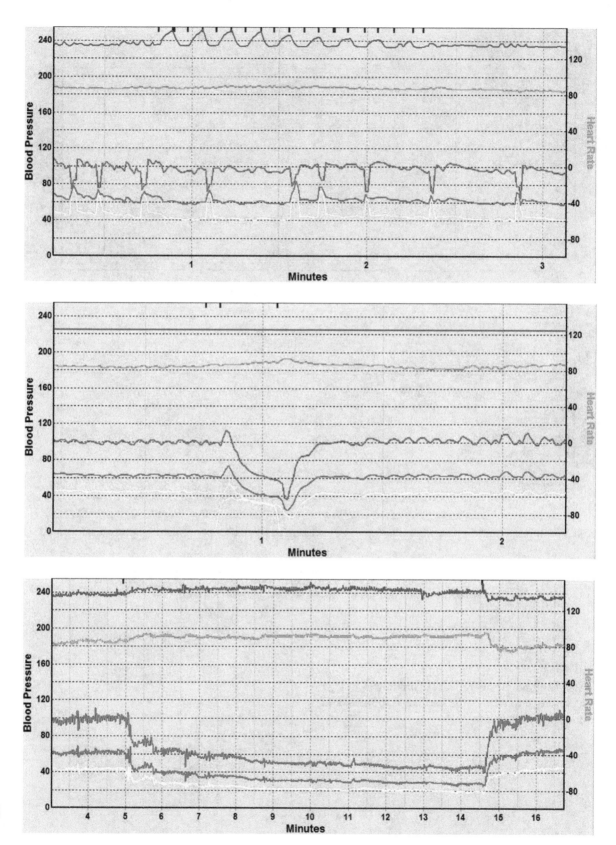

Vignette 14

Anxiety: the pattern is very similar to hyperadrenergic POTS, but here note that the maximal heart rate value during tilt occurs immediately upon tilt-up with subsequent decline, while in POTS the opposite is true.

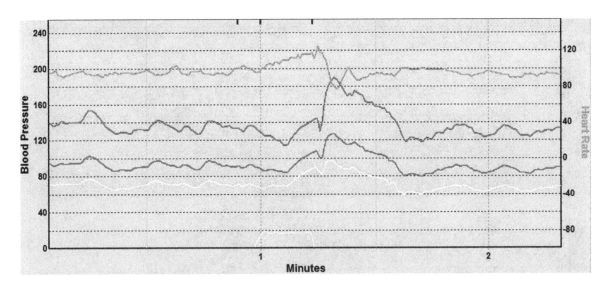

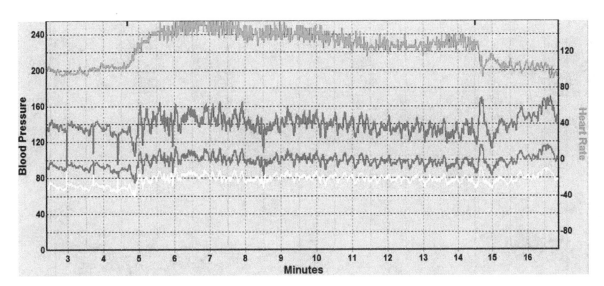

Vignette 15

Patient with severe, long-standing autonomic failure. Note the marked supine hypertension that develops over time to compensate for the orthostatic hypotension. Patients like this tolerate high BP likely due to expanded cerebral autoregulation curve. Treated too aggressively their BP would result in worsening symptoms of OH. The best management is by elevating their bed head and using short-acting antihypertensive agents at night, but refraining from using them during the day.

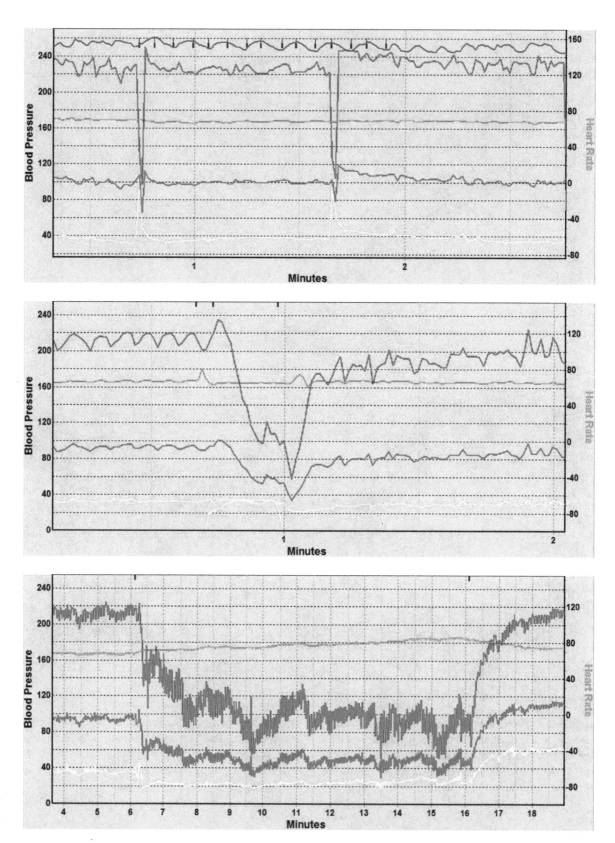

Vignette 16

Patient with tetraplegia. Heart rate responses to DB were still relatively preserved. His blood pressure profile during Valsalva shows absence of late phase II recovery and phase IV overshoot as well as prolonged recovery time. Heart rate response is slow and inadequate. Tilt in the same subject shows severe orthostatic hypotension with almost absent cardiac responses. Sweat responses in the same patient. Responses are normal proximally, absent in the foot.

(16.1a)

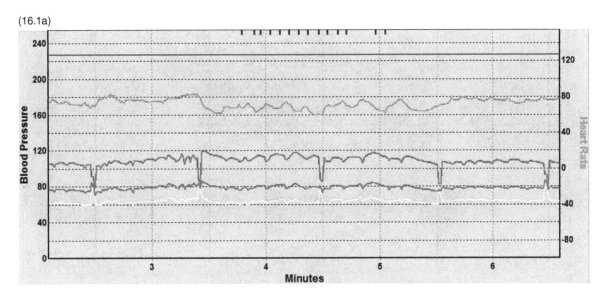

(16.1b)

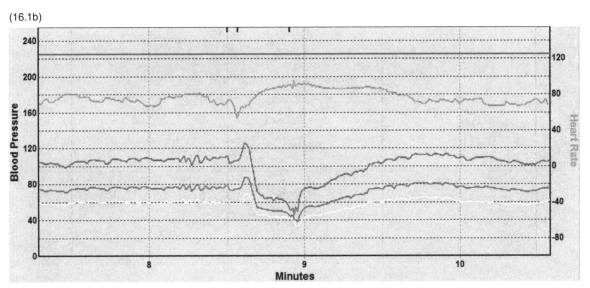

Vignettes

(16.1c)

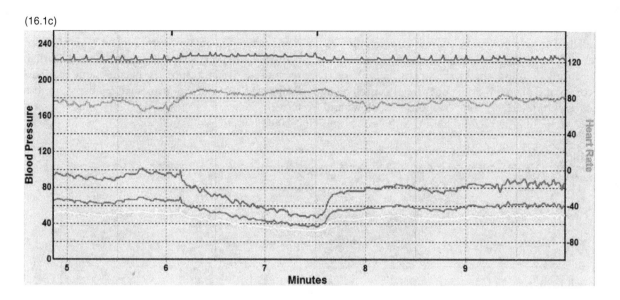

(16.1d)

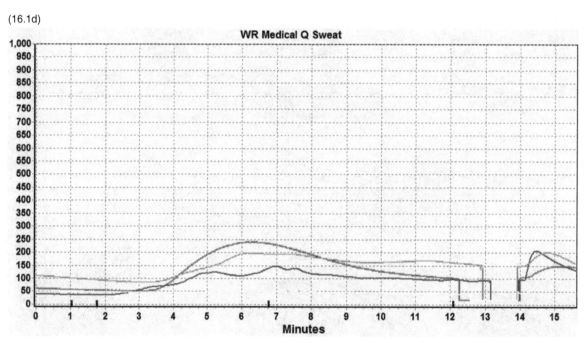

Vignette 17

High sympathetic outflow (examples each showing DB and VM): resting tachycardia prevents normal heart rate response during deep breathing. During Valsalva, as the stimulus is stronger, vagal modulation becomes evident particularly during phase IV.

(17.1a)

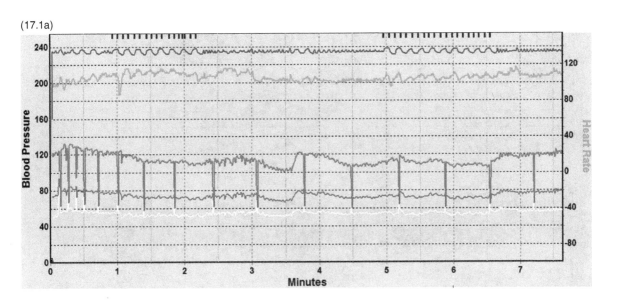

(17.1b)

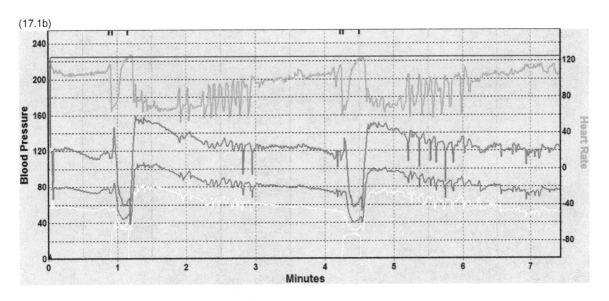

(17.2a)

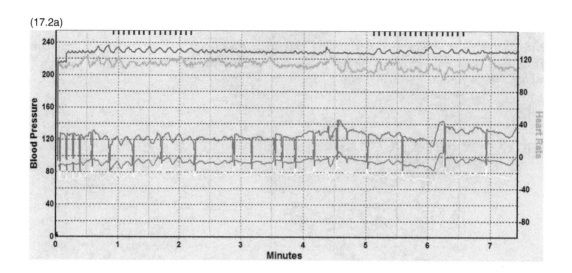

(17.2b)

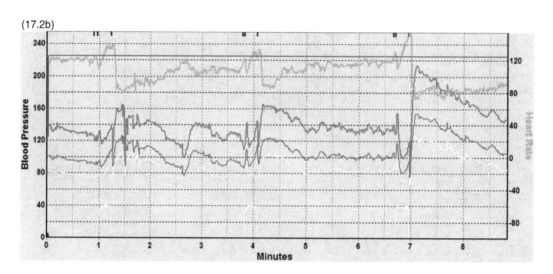

(17.3a)

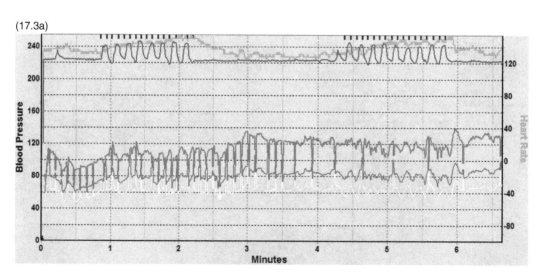

(17.3b)

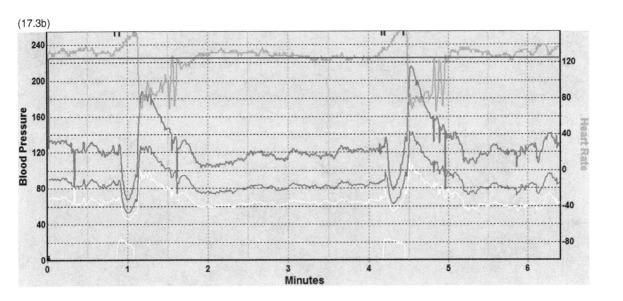

(17.4a)

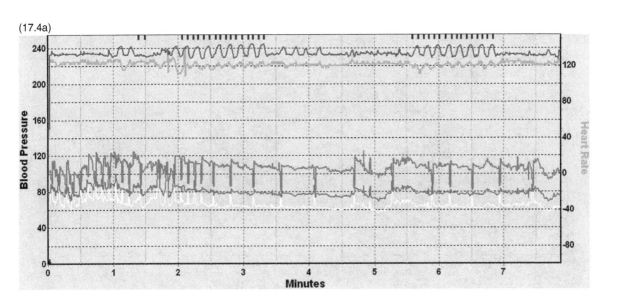

(17.4b)

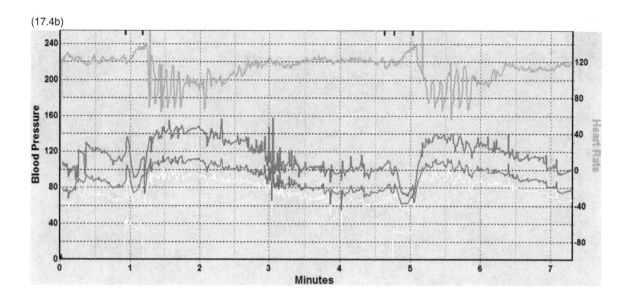

(17.5a)

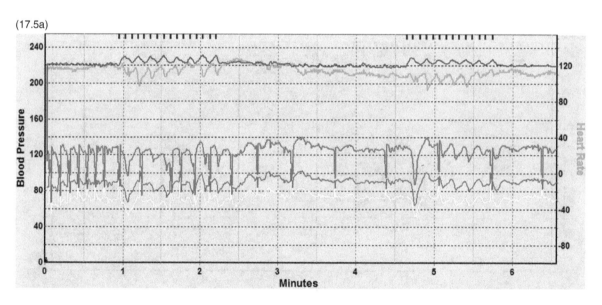

(17.5b)

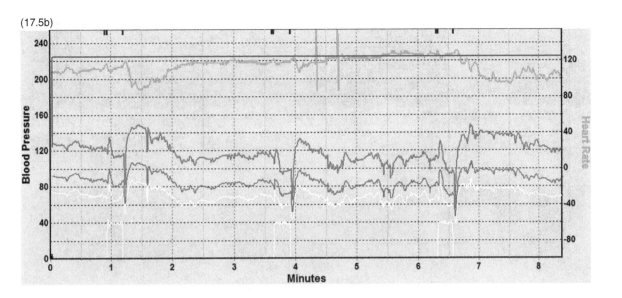

Vignette 18

Incidental finding: spontaneous Cheyne–Stokes breathing observed during baseline before tilt in a patient with neurodegenerative disorder.

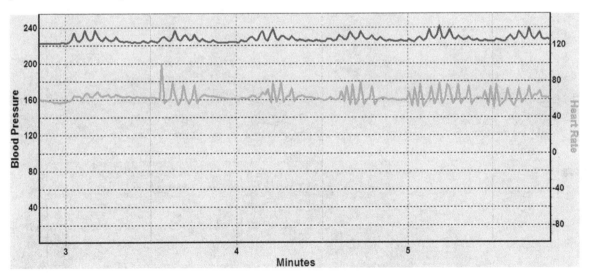

Vignette 19

Diabetic autonomic neuropathy: Heart rate response to deep breathing is essentially absent, and to the Valsalva maneuver is reduced while vasomotor function is still preserved. QSART shows absent (distal leg and foot) or markedly reduced (proximal leg) sweat responses in the lower limb. In this patient the pattern of involvement is thus one mainly of cholinergic failure.

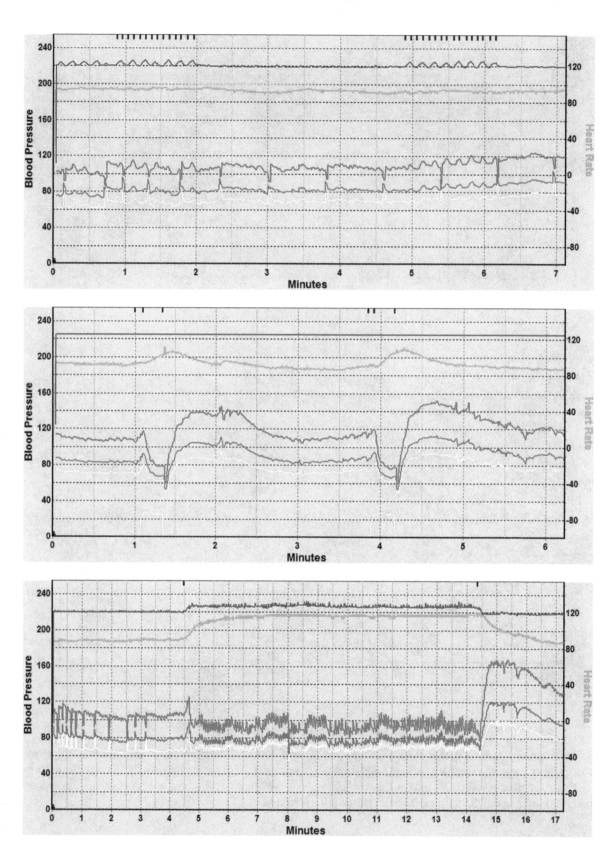

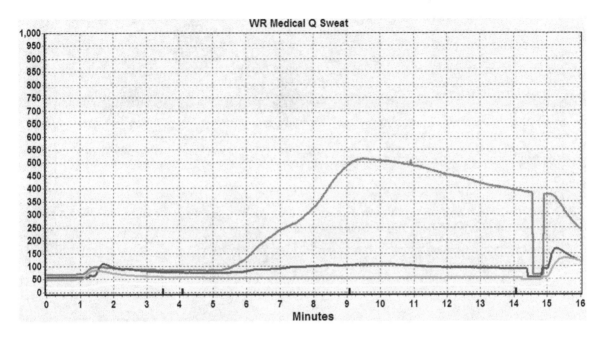

Vignette 20

A case of HIV: autonomic involvement is usually mild in HIV-related neuropathy, as in this example: there is modest cardiovagal, vasomotor, and length-dependent sudomotor dysfunction.

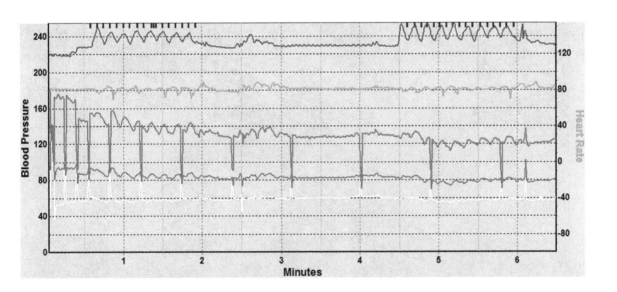

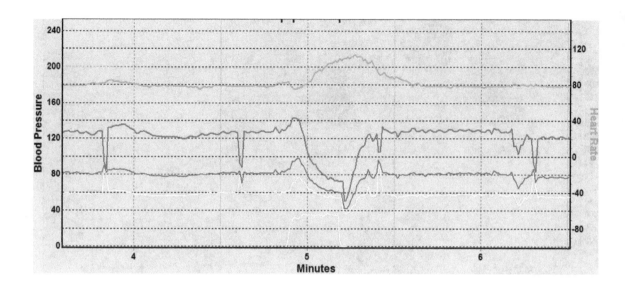

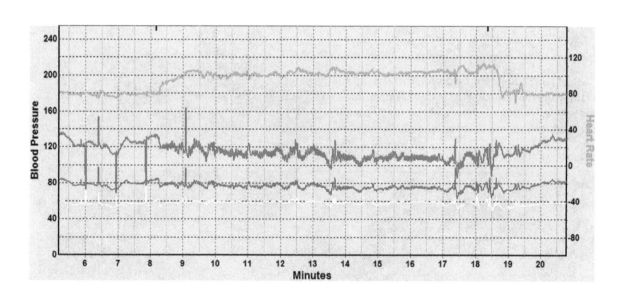

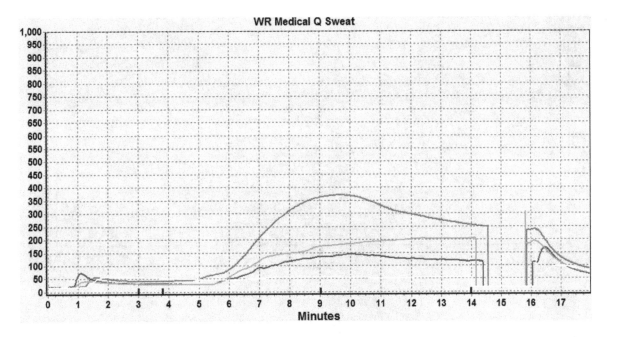

Vignette 21

A patient with Guillain-Barré and prominent autonomic, mainly vasomotor, failure. The patient became presyncopal after less than a minute of tilt. The blood pressure profile during Valsalva shows complete absence of late phase II and IV and prolonged recovery time. Cardiac response is still relatively preserved. QSART was absent in the lower limb.

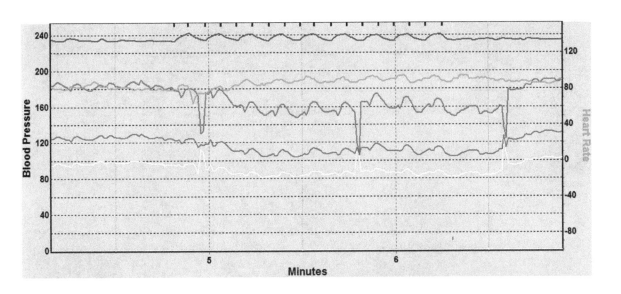

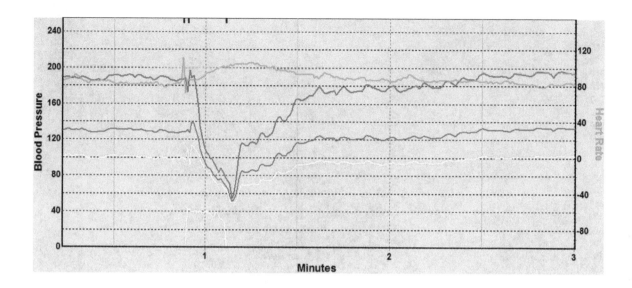

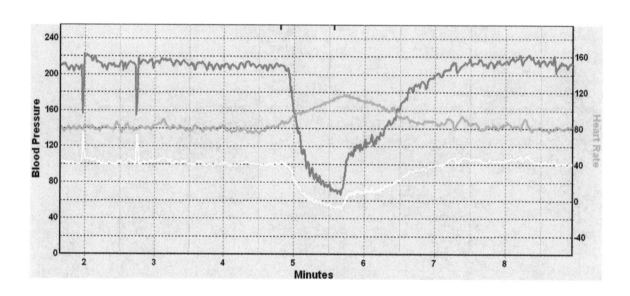

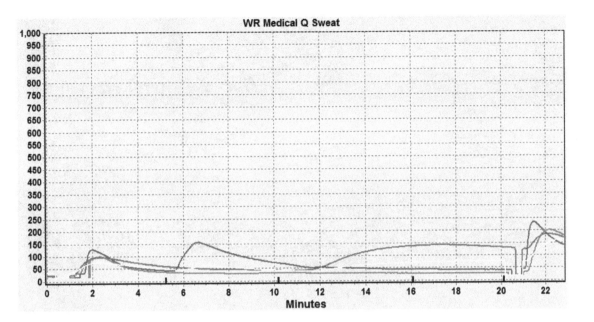

Vignette 22

Effect of gasp before Valsalva: note the marked drop in heart rate at the start of the maneuver. As a con-sequence of that, the Valsalva ratio may be spuriously reduced.

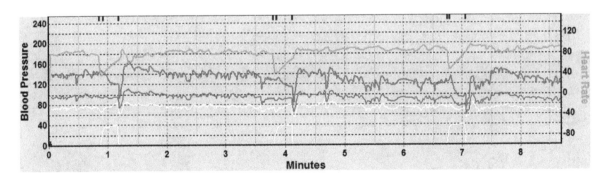

Vignette 23

A series of Valsalva maneuvers performed supine and with bed tilted at 20 and 30 degrees in a normal subject who had a square wave blood pressure response. Note that with tilting of the bed the profile changes and the phases are clearly recognizable.

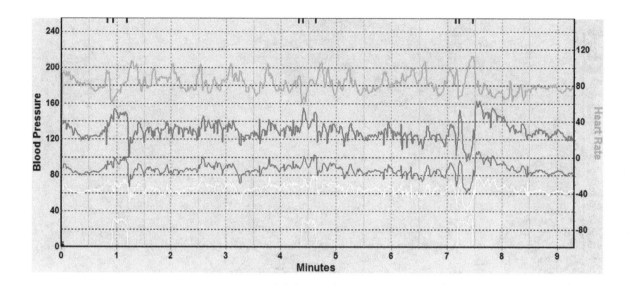

Vignette 24

In contrast, series in a patient with congestive heart failure: the "square-wave" blood pressure profile does not change with slight tilting (20 and 30 degrees respectively for the second and third maneuvers). This is abnormal and is due to elevated left ventricle end-diastolic pressure.

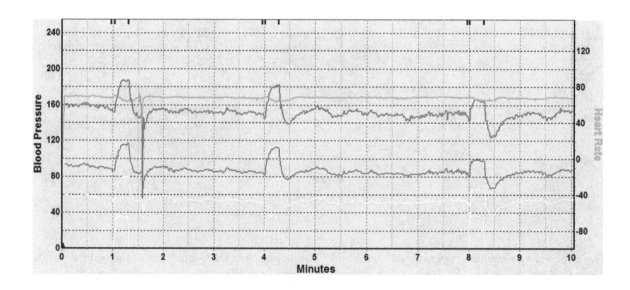

Vignette 25

Two cases of pure autonomic failure: the second case (25.2a–d) is more advanced, but in both the global dysfunction can be clearly seen, with impaired post-ganglionic sudomotor responses, cardiovagal and sympathetic failure, manifesting as reduced cardiac responses, abnormal Valsalva profile, and orthostatic hypotension.

(25.1a)

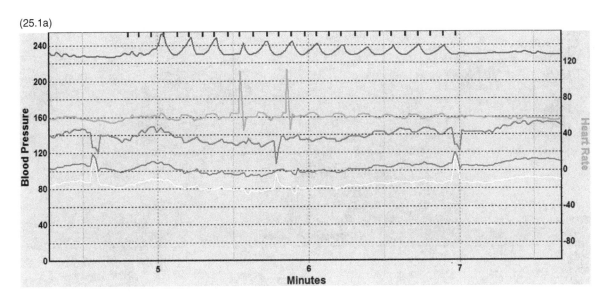

(25.1b)

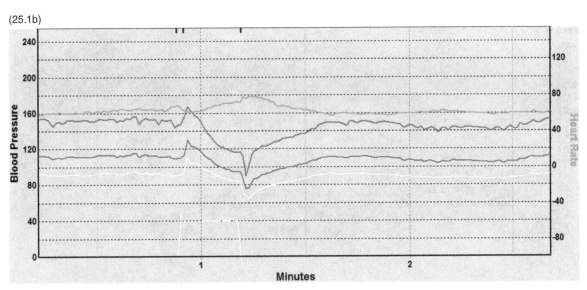

Vignettes

(25.1c)

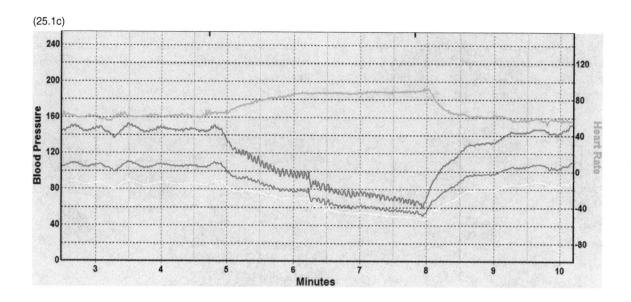

(25.1d)

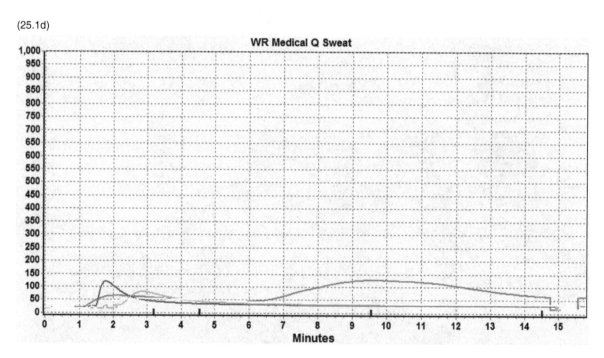

152

(25.2a)

(25.2b)

(25.2c)

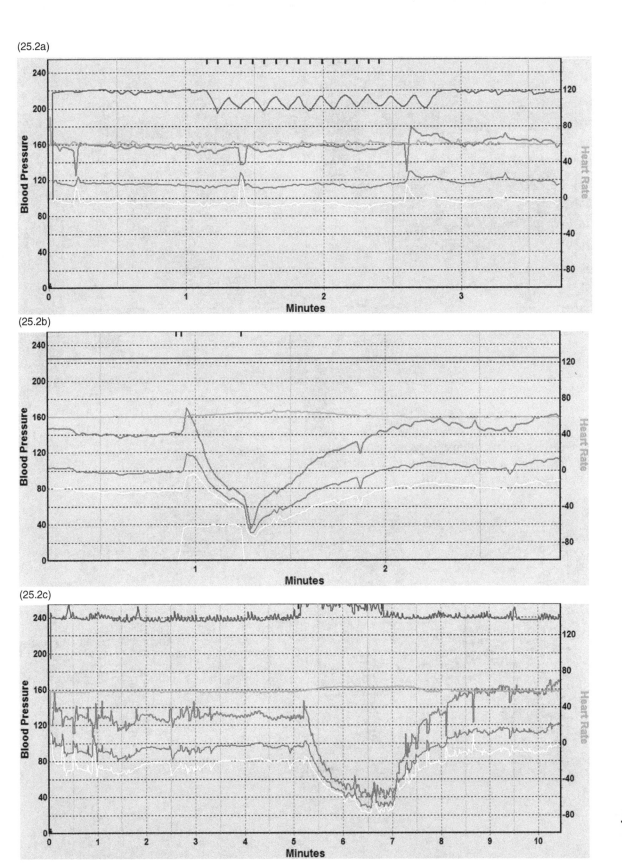

(25.2d)

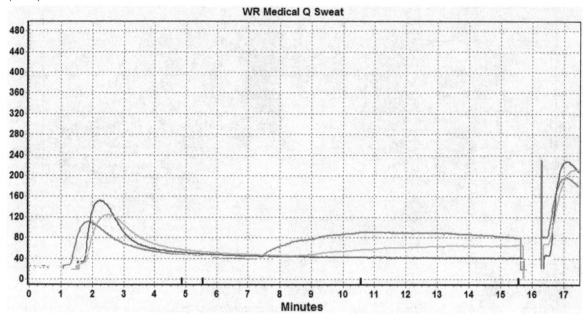

Vignette 26

Brief episode of arrhythmia triggered by Valsalva maneuver. This is not uncommon, particularly in the young and again in the elderly.

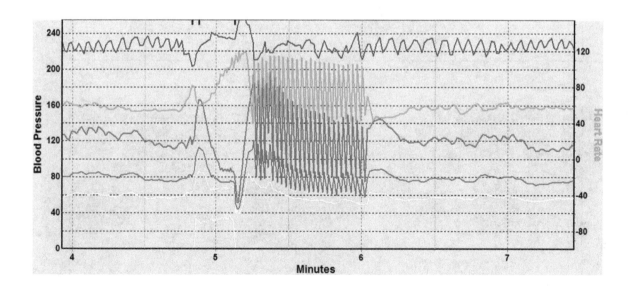

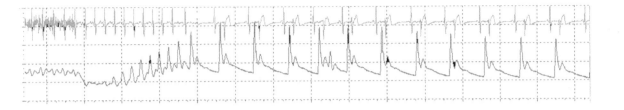

Vignette 27

Early, transient hypotension after tilt-up (three cases). This is commonly seen in patients treated with antihypertensive medications, in hypovolemia or severe deconditioning.

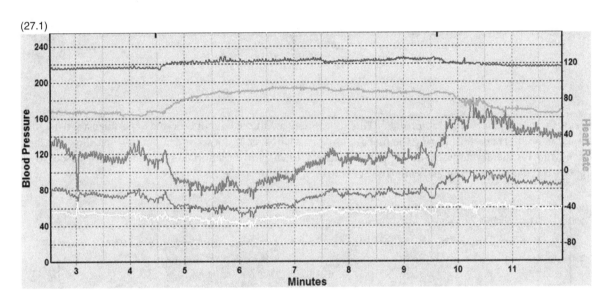

(27.1)

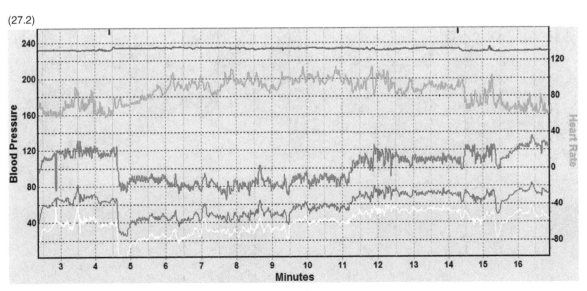

(27.2)

(27.3)

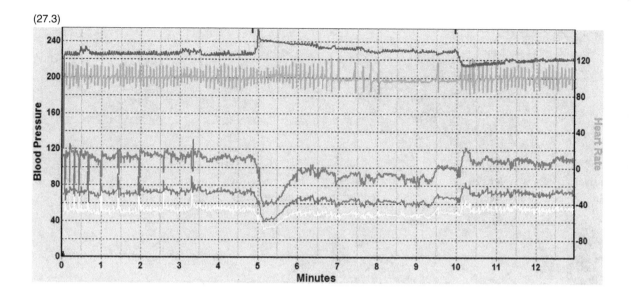

Vignette 28

Spuriously abnormal Valsalva profile. This was caused by too short an effort during the first attempt, not allowing for the development of late phase II. An attentive technician noticed it and with some encour-agement the patient was able to perform a satisfactory maneuver at the second attempt, when she was asked to sustain the effort longer but allowed to do so at lower pressure.

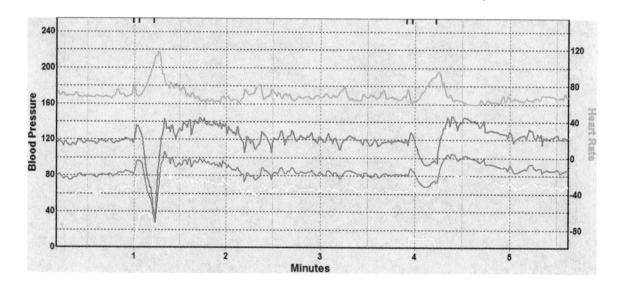

Vignette 29

Patient interrupted briefly the expiratory effort during Valsalva, generating a dip in heart rate and a small rise in blood pressure during phase II.

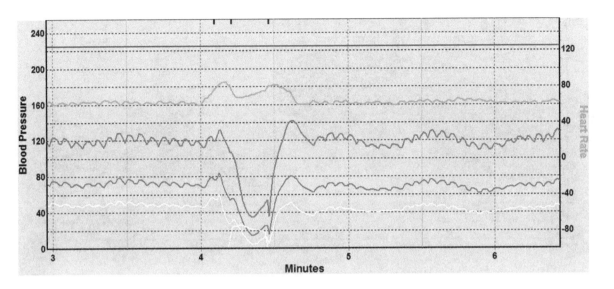

Vignette 30

Medication effect: beta blocker blunted cardioacceleration during Valsalva, prolonged the blood pressure recovery time and abolished phase IV overshoot.

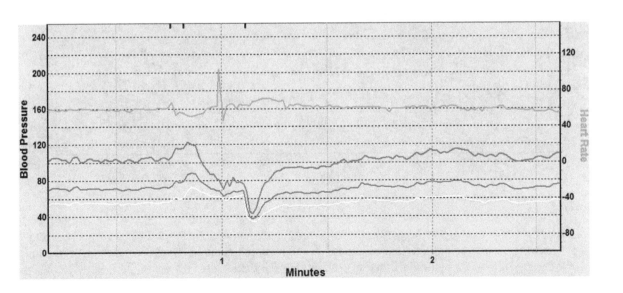

Vignette 31

Patient with limited autonomic neuropathy with selective involvement of vasomotor fibers. Note during Valsalva the absence of late phase II, prolonged blood pressure recovery time, and attenuated phase IV. During tilt, the patient had orthostatic hypotension. Cardiac response was valid during both tests.

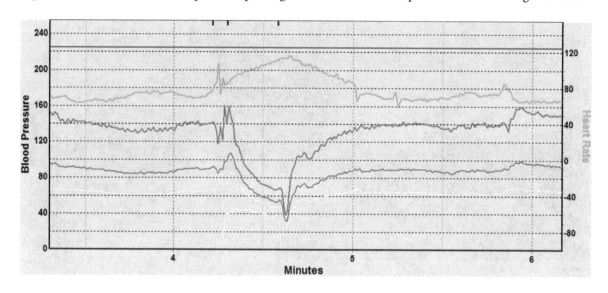

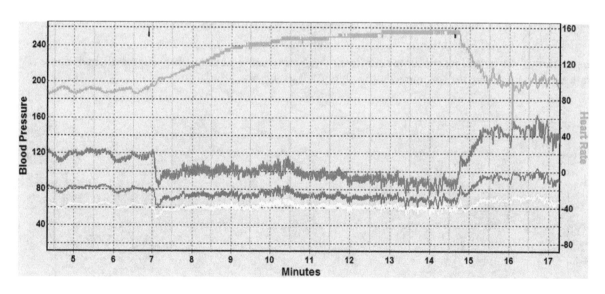

Vignette 32

Deep breathing in patient with autonomic neuropathy. The response was actually markedly reduced, but an episode of arrhythmia made it look like a normal one. Caution should be paid to ECG tracings in such cases.

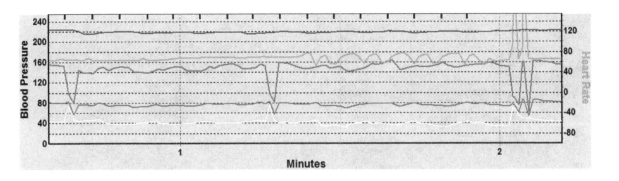

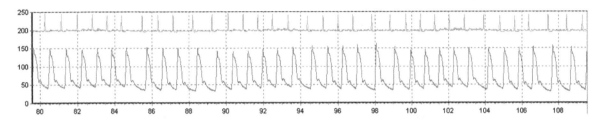

Vignette 33

During the study, while obtaining baseline, a patient experienced a brief anxiety attack with hyperventilation and tachycardia.

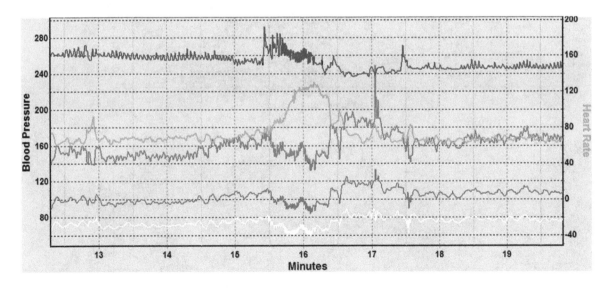

Vignette 34

Pacemaker effect series: by preventing the heart rate from dropping below the set value, pacemakers may reduce the amplitude of cardiac responses both on deep breathing (34.1–2) and Valsalva maneuver (34.3–4).

159

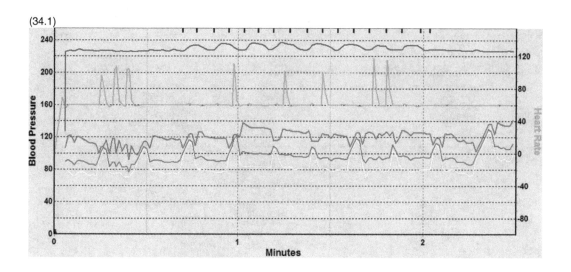

(34.1)

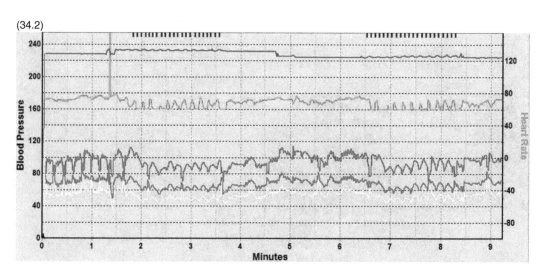

(34.2)

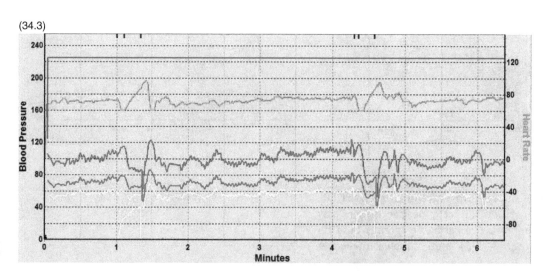

(34.3)

(34.4)

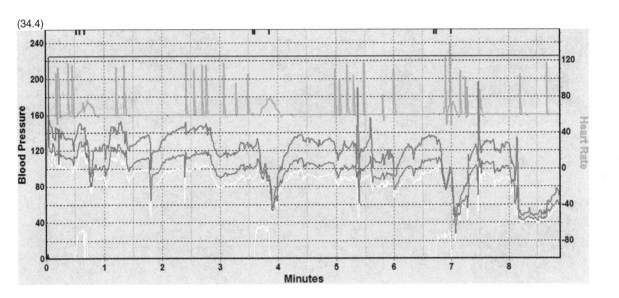

Vignette 35

Vasodepressor syncope: the decline in blood pressure
is accompanied by a spike in heart rate.

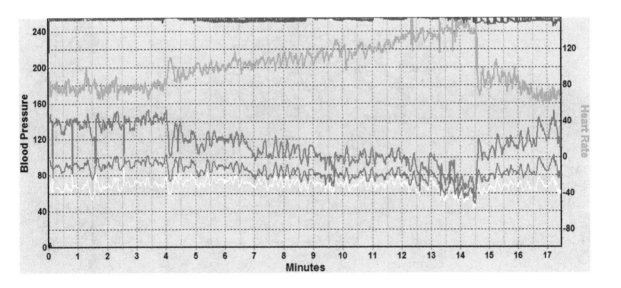

Vignette 36

Vasovagal syncope: in this case both heart rate and
blood pressure drop simultaneously.

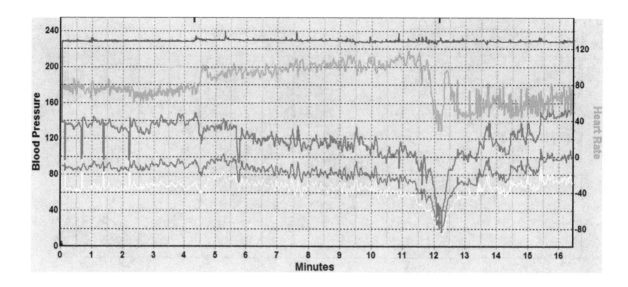

Vignette 37

Patient with atrial fibrillation. Occasionally, even if a precise value cannot be calculated, qualitatively the ability to appropriately modulate the heart rate during Valsalva can be appreciated.

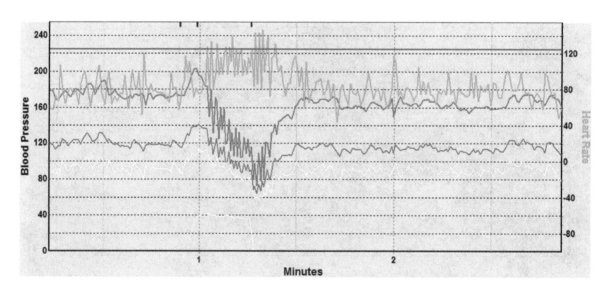

Vignette 38

QSART response asymmetry in a patient with CRPS. The yellow and blue tracings are from the right limb, the red and green from the left. The affected limb may sweat more or less than the contralateral. In this case, the left limb was the painful one.

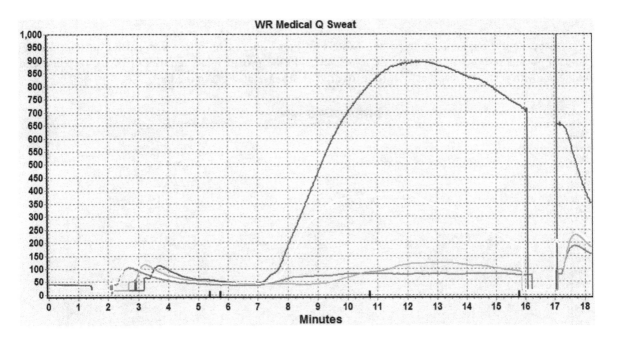

Vignette 39

Patient with diabetic length-dependent neuropathy. There was absent distal sweat while at the two proximal sites there was persistent sweat activity (instead of tapering off at the end of the stimulation, the response actually increases). This can represent compensatory response, early denervation supersensitivity or terminals irritability.

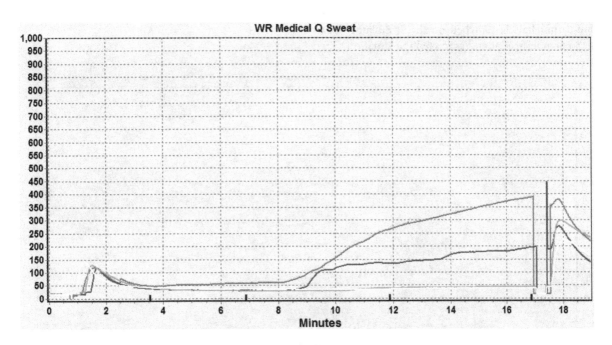

Vignette 40

Length-dependent peripheral neuropathy. QSART showed a normal response in the forearm, a normal volume but with persistent sweat activity (due to early small fiber involvement with partial supersensitivity) in the proximal leg, reduced distal leg response and absence of sweat in the foot.

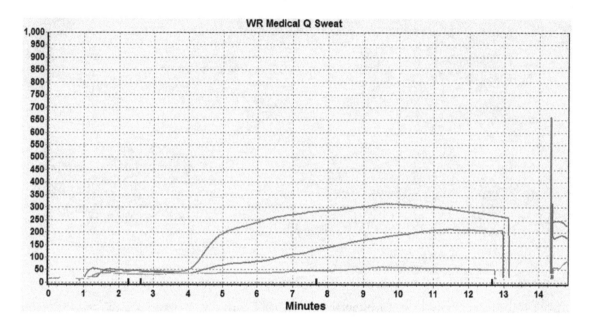

Vignette 41

The apparent delay in sweat responses was actually due to not having switched on the stimulator. One technician noticed it and corrected the situation.

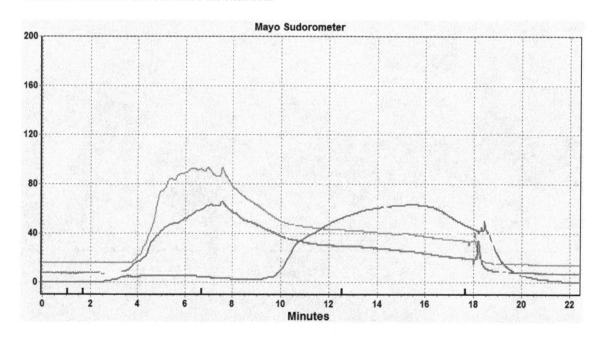

Vignette 42

QSART in a patient with neuropathic pain and allodynia: the ultra-short latency is due to allodynia triggering a somato-sympathetic response.

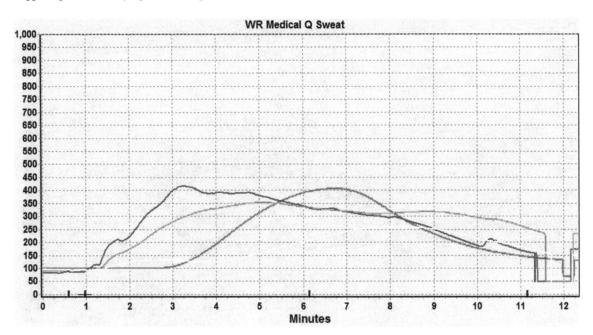

Vignette 43

Resting sweat detected in a patient with severe pruritus before QSART (a). (b) Another example of resting sweat. This can be seen in normal subjects: anxiety, pain may exacerbate it. In these cases adequate time should be allowed before starting the stimulation in order to have a reliable baseline.

(a)

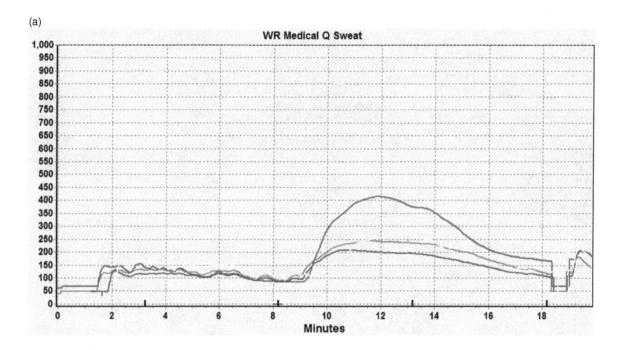

(b)

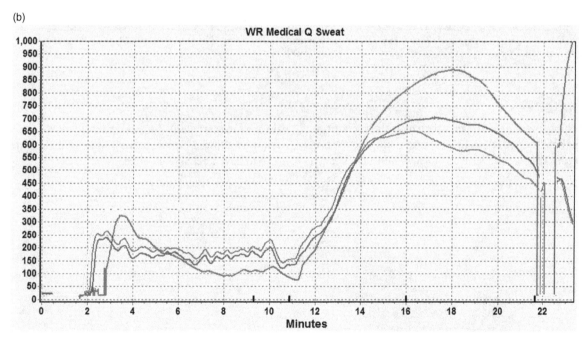

Vignette 44

Anticholinergic effect on sweat responses (a). After withholding the medication, the test normalized (b). However, if patient has been on such agents for a long time, sweat glands may atrophy and thus sweat production may remain low.

(a)

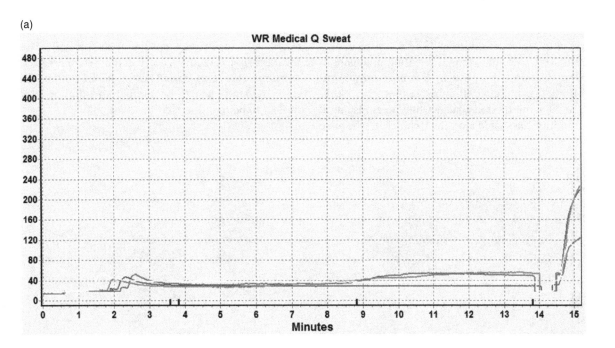

(b)

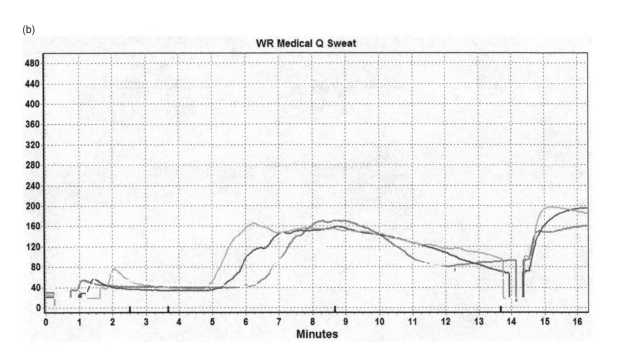

Vignette 45

Three examples of leak during QSART due to sudden twitch at the foot site (arrows) resulting in apparent increase in sweat response in the final minute of recording (a), and after stimulus was turned off (b). The sudden, unexpected change while sweat response was diminishing should alert the technician, who also noted the sudden foot movement in this case. The third example (c) showed a leak in the system detected as soon as recording started but before the iontophoresis. The study had to be aborted and the capsules needed to be repositioned.

(a)

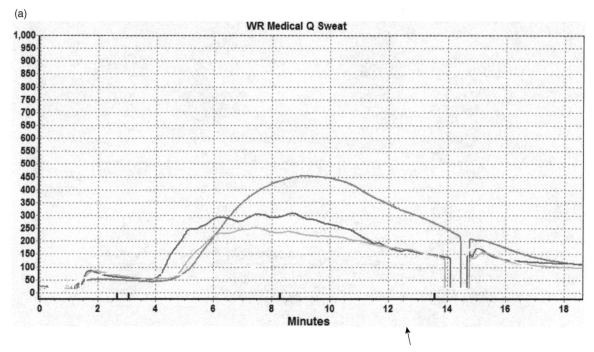

(b)

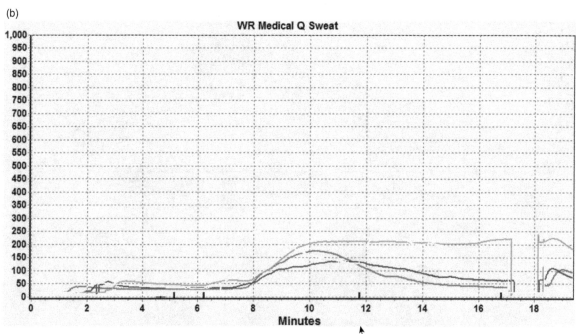

(c)

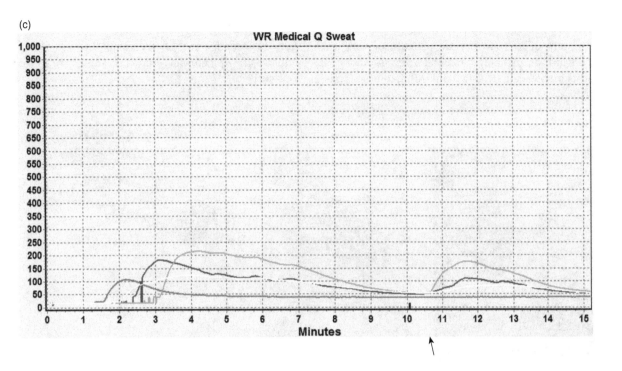

Vignette 46

Examples of TST in diabetic patients showing the spectrum of pathology ranging from lumbosacral radiculoplexopathy, distal and more diffuse small fiber neuropathy, truncal radiculopathy, and global anhidrosis. (A normal study is shown first for comparison.)

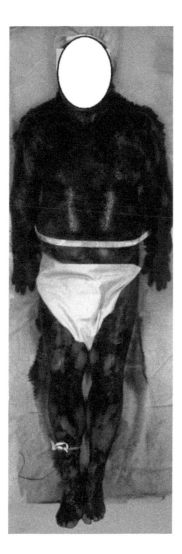

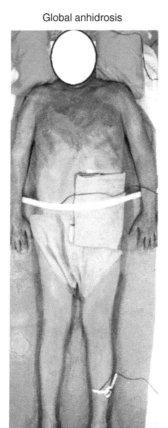

Global anhidrosis

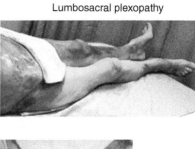

Lumbosacral plexopathy

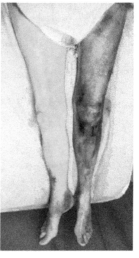

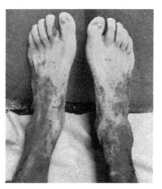

Distal small
fiber neuropathy

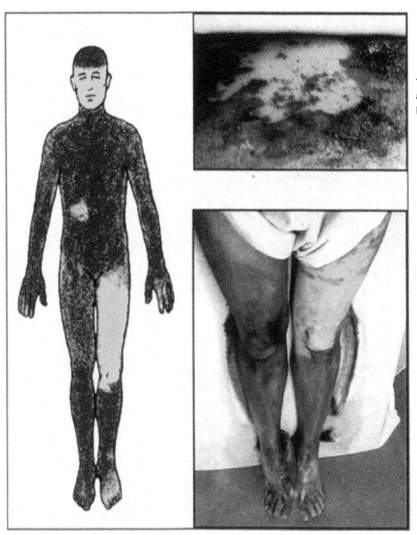

Thoracic radiculopathy
and lumbosacral
plexopathy

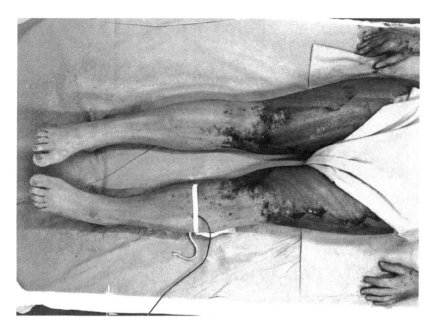

Length-dependent and patchy, diffuse neuropathy

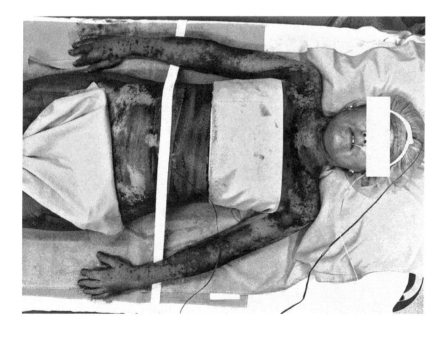

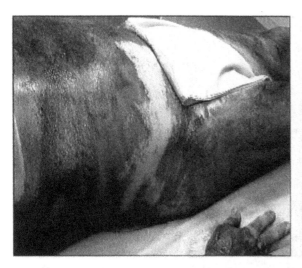

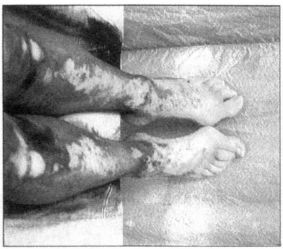

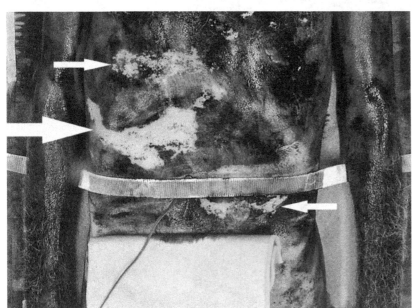

Thoracic radiculopathy
and distal small
fiber neuropathy

Vignette 47

Case of gustatory sweating: note the purple stain (indicating sweat) before (a) and after eating (b).

(47.1a)

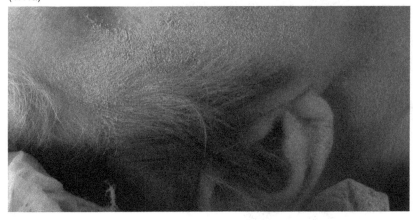

(47.1b)

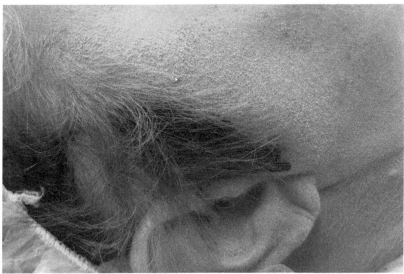

Vignette 48

Patient with a thoracic cord mass lesion, who presented with increased sweating in the thoracic dermatome corresponding to the level of the lesion. Images before and after tumor removal, which resulted in anhidrosis of the left trunk.

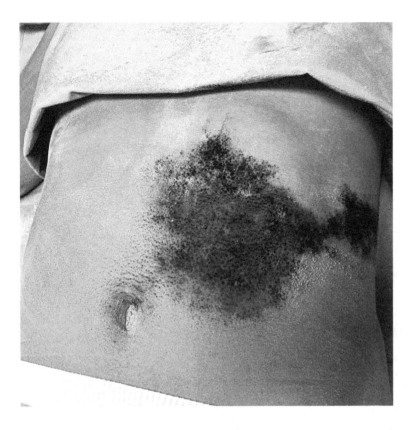

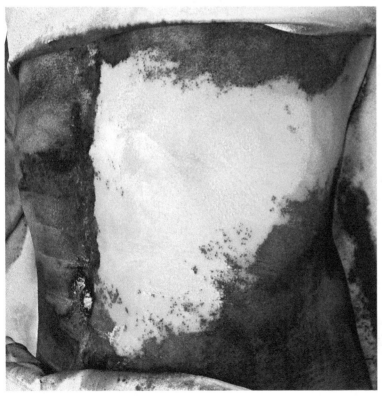

Vignette 49

TST series in a patient with cord AVM causing irritation of the sympathetic pathways. He began to sweat on the left, where the lesion was.

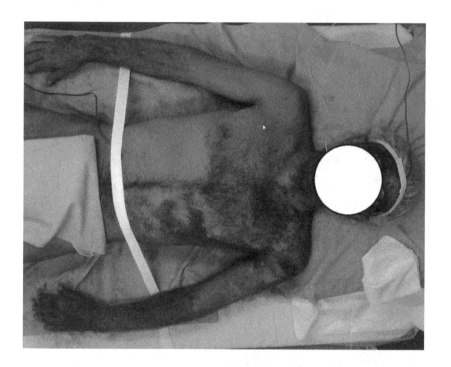

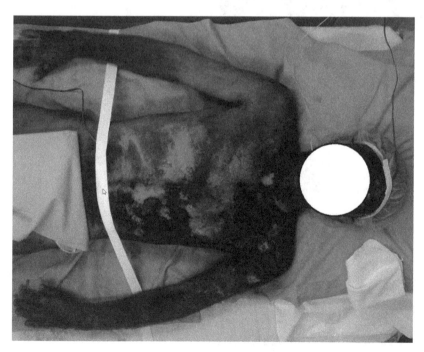

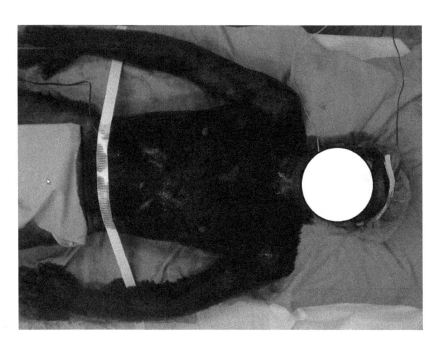

Vignette 50

Patient with MSA. Note the global anhidrosis with the unique distal preservation, commonly seen in central autonomic disorders.

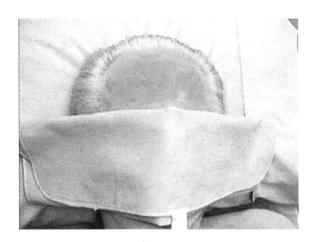

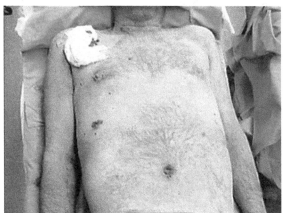

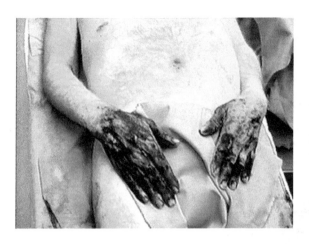

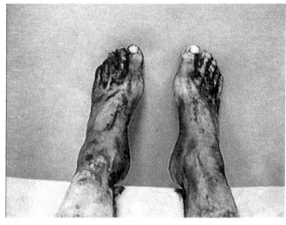

Vignette 51
Acral hyperhidrosis (pre-heat images).

Vignette 52
Postsympathectomy study.

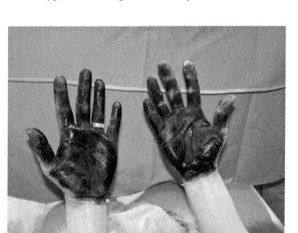

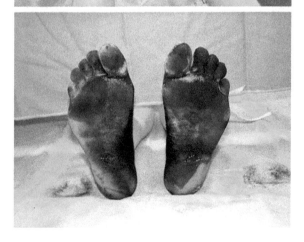

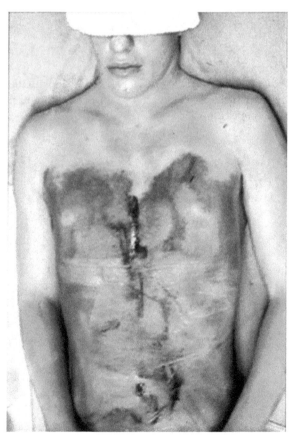

Vignette 53

Anhidrosis over the forehead can be seen in cluster headache and in migraine sufferers. It is also seen after Botox injection for migraine treatment or cosmetic use.

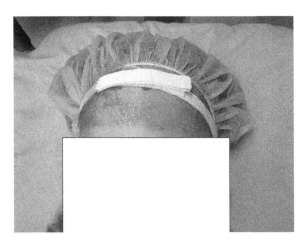

Vignette 55

Distal anhidrosis in patient with burning feet and distal small fiber neuropathy.

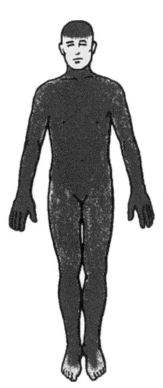

Vignette 54

An example of left lower limb anhidrosis, due to plexopathy in this case.

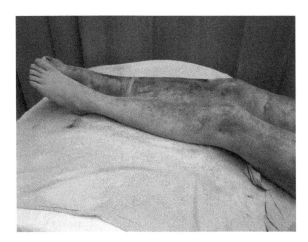

Vignette 56

Focal loss of sweating in area of prior burn injury.

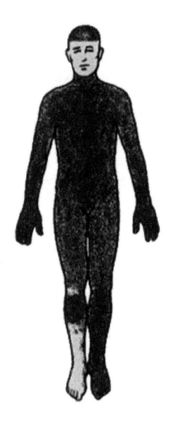

Recommended reading

Benarroch, E.E. (2006). *Basic Neurosciences with Clinical Applications*. Philadelphia, PA: Butterworth Heinemann/ Elsevier.

Benarroch, E.E. (2014). *Autonomic Neurology*. New York, NY: Oxford University Press.

Low, P.A. and Benarroch, E.E. (eds) (2008). *Clinical Autonomic Disorders* (3rd edn). Philadelphia, PA: Lippincott, Williams & Wilkins.

Robertson, D., Biaggioni, I., Burnstock, G., Low, P.A. and Paton, J.F.R. (eds) (2012). *BiagPrimer of the Autonomic Nervous System* (3rd edn). San Diego, CA: Elsevier.

Index

Figures are noted in bold typeface.

CPSIA information can be obtained
at www.ICGtesting.com
Printed in the USA
LVHW060219240421
685369LV00009B/306